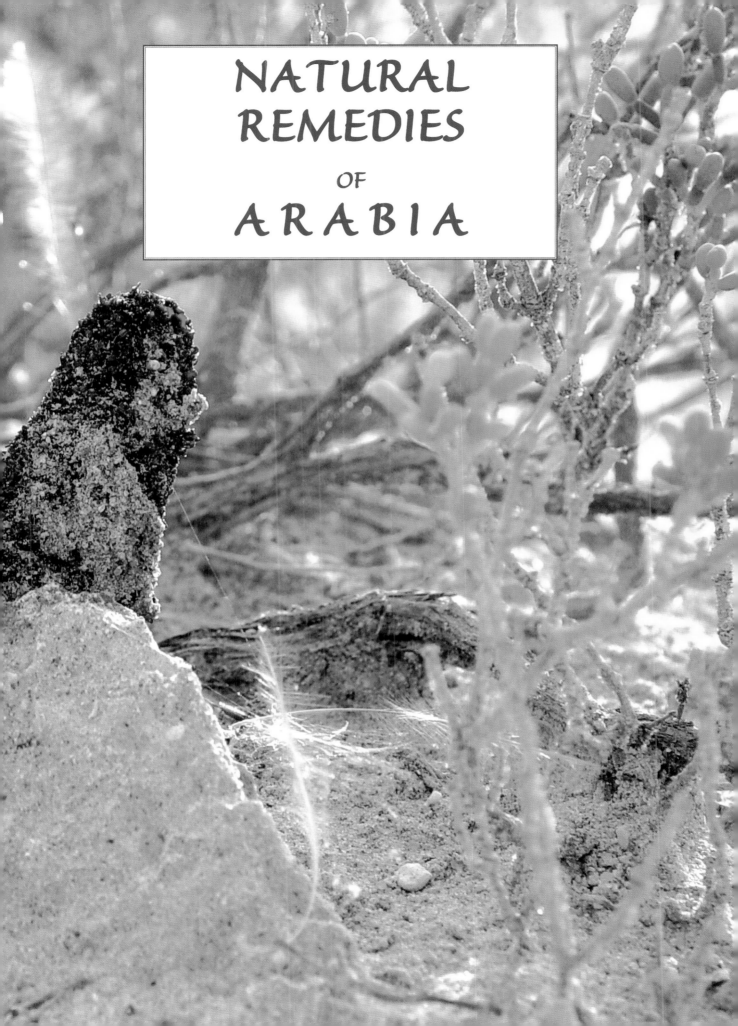

NATURAL
REMEDIES
OF
ARABIA

Natural Remedies of Arabia
published by
Stacey International
128 Kensington Church Street
London W8 4BH
Tel: +44 (0)20 7221 7166 Fax: +44 (0)20 7792 9288
E-mail: enquiries@stacey-international.co.uk
Website: www.stacey-international.co.uk

with
Al-Turath
PO Box 68200
Riyadh 11527
The Kingdom of Saudi Arabia
E-mail: al-turath@al.turath.com
Website: www.al-turath.com
Tel: +9661 980 7710
Fax: +9661 980 7708

ISBN: 1-905299-02-8

CIP Data: A catalogue record for this book is available from the British Library

Design: Kitty Carruthers
Printing & Binding: SNP Leefung, China

Photographic credits:
Principal photographer Donna Pepperdine

Stephen L. Brundage/Saudi Aramco: 28, 42, 46, 74, 98, 102(b), 112, 113, 122(t), 146(2), 150(2);
Linda Lebling: 14, 39, 84(2), 128(2), 186, 206; John J. S. Burton/Saudi Aramco (*Cultivated
Outdoor Plants of Saudi Aramco)*: 11, 38, 106, 130, 155, 157, 164; Faleh S. Khashram: 107, 108,
134(2), 162; Faisal I. Al Dossary/Saudi Aramco: 47, 132(b), 138(b), 180, 197; Saudi Aramco: 118,
121; N. L. Britton & A. Brown (*Illustrated Flora of the Northern States and Canada*, 1913)
courtesy of Kentucky Native Plant Society, scanned by Omnitek Inc.: 99, 117; Kristie
Burns/*Saudi Aramco World*/PADIA: 177; Saad M. Haboob: 79; James P Mandaville (*Flora of
Eastern Saudi Arabia)*: 132(t)

Publication of this work has been made possible
with the support of Saudi Aramco

ارامكو السعودية
Saudi Aramco

NATURAL
REMEDIES
OF
ARABIA

Robert W.
LEBLING
&
Donna
PEPPERDINE, MH

AL - TURATH / STACEY INTERNATIONAL

CONTENTS

ACKNOWLEDGEMENTS

We, the authors thank the many families of Arabia who generously shared knowledge of herbal traditions, past and present. We gratefully acknowledge:

Those who reviewed the remedies contributed from the different regions of the Arabian Peninsula and provided additional detail:

Haya S. Al-Issa (Najd, Central Province)
Munirah K. Al-Suwailem (Najd, Central Province)
Faisal K. Al-Suwailem (Najd, Central Province)
Quriyan M. Al-Hajri, Supervisor, Inspection Unit, Wellsites Division, Drilling and Workover Services, Saudi Aramco ('Ain Dar, Eastern Province)
Hamsa Mathker Al-Hajri ('Ain Dar, Eastern Province)
Yahya Al-Zaid, Vice President, Sales and Marketing, Saudi Aramco (Hail, Northern Province)
Aisha Kay, EFL Teacher/Career Counsellor, Saudi Aramco (Dhahran, Eastern Province)
Maryam Al-Moalem, Lactation Education Specialist, Saudi Aramco (Qatif, Eastern Province)
Munira Al-Ashgar (Dhahran, Eastern Province)
Muhammad A. Tahlawi, Saudi Aramco Affairs, Saudi Aramco (Dhahran, Eastern Province)
Dr. Jabber Salem Mossa Al-Kahtani, Professor and Chairman of the Department of Pharmacognosy, King Saud University (Abha, Southern Province)

Those who helped us locate out-of-the-way herb shops:

Colin Hewitt, Management Training Consultant, Saudi Aramco (Dhahran, Eastern Province)
Mahdi Al-Jamed (Qatif, Eastern Province)
Mustafa A. Jalali, Vice President, Saudi Aramco Affairs, Saudi Aramco (Jeddah, Western Province)

Those who assisted with questionnaire distribution and translations:

Haifa Al-Mansour, English Language Trainer, Saudi Aramco (al-Hasa, Eastern Province)
Abeer Zaki, English Language Trainer, Saudi Aramco (Makkah, Western Province)
Eman Bukhamsin (al-Hasa, Eastern Province)
June Titheridge (United Arab Emirates)

Those who offered constant support, inspiration and encouragement:

Colin Hewitt, Management Training Consultant, Saudi Aramco
Aisha Kay, EFL Teacher/Career Counsellor, Saudi Aramco
Beverly Pepperdine (Saudi Aramco retiree 1954-1959, 1977-1991)
Nasser A. Al-Nafisee, Manager, Public Relations, Saudi Aramco
Linda Lebling, Nature Photographer (Saudi Arabia resident 1994-5)

INTRODUCTION.

Whether you are in Doha, Dubai, Manama, Salalah, Jeddah or an obscure country village, when you step into an herbal medicine shop or wander through the traditional *suqs*, you will find vendors of oils, herbs, spices, bark, twigs, rocks and salt intended for culinary, cosmetic or medicinal purposes.

As you gaze at the piles of twisted bark or the varied combinations of dried flowers, you may wonder:

> What are these products?
> Where do they come from?
> How are they used locally?

This book will help you to recognize the varied offerings of the herb shops and markets and even impress local vendors as you request, with knowledge and confidence, a half kilo of *habba sawda* or a small bag of *rumman*.

These fascinating items whisper tales of the ancient trade routes, for many still come to Arabia from India, China, Indonesia, Egypt, Syria and other exotic locations, and are distributed across the Peninsula through existing commercial networks. Others are harvested locally, some under harsh desert conditions, and have their own fascinating stories to tell.

The people of the Arabian Peninsula have, for centuries, combined goods obtained by trade and bartering with a prudent use of local plants and have developed a rich heritage of folk medicine.

Many of the natural remedies presented in this book are the result of a questionnaire distributed throughout the Arabian Peninsula in early 2002. The questionnaire, printed in both Arabic and English, asked families to explain how they, as well as their mothers and grandmothers, use various herbs, spices and other substances in natural healing. It also requested specific remedies for conditions such as headaches, coughs and colds, sore throats, hair loss, general fatigue, childbirth, etc. We present their generous responses which have helped to unlock many of the mysteries of local medicinal herb shops and reveal unique insights into the natural remedies of Arabia.

R.W.L. and D.P.

The remedies presented in the following pages have been provided by people of the Arabian peninsula, in Saudi Arabia, Bahrain, Yemen, Oman and the United Arab Emirates. They represent past and present usage of natural substances used in folk healing. Following each remedy is the location of the family origin of the person sharing the remedy. The provinces of The Kingdom of Saudi Arabia are referred to as Eastern KSA, Northern KSA, etc.

NATURAL REMEDIES

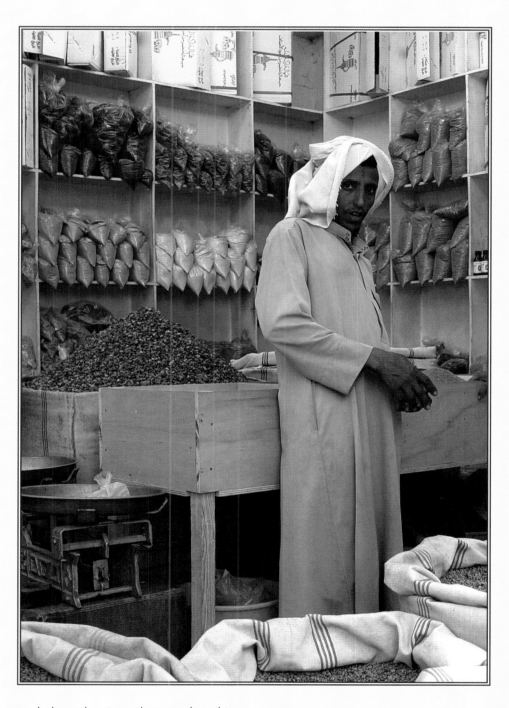

Herb shop, Khamis Mushayt, Saudi Arabia.

ALOE
Aloe vera
Aloeaceae (Aloe) Family
Arabic: *sabir, sabr, subaar*

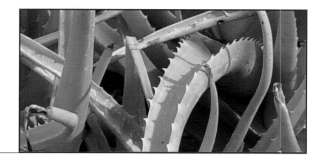

This remarkable and well-known succulent appears to have originated in eastern Africa and then spread to Arabia and beyond. Its medicinal qualities were recognized quite early – it has been used to treat burns since ancient times – but the plant also had other qualities which some might call spiritual.

On his celebrated pilgrimage to Makkah and Madinah in 1853, British adventurer Sir Richard Burton saw some parched aloe plants growing in Jannat al-Ma'ala, the sacred cemetery of Makkah, and wrote:

The Aloe here, as in Egypt, is hung, like the dried crocodile, over houses as a talisman against evil spirits. [Swiss traveller Johann L.] Burckhardt assigns, as a motive for it being planted in graveyards, that its name Saber denotes the patience with which the believer awaits the Last Day. And [the British anthropologist Edward] Lane remarks, 'The Aloe thus hung (over the door), without earth and water, will live for several years, and even blossom: hence it is called Saber, which signifies patience.'

HOW TO USE

To access aloe gel, cut along the outer edges of the leaf and peel back the skin to collect the thick mucilaginous gel inside. Aloe gel naturally oozes from a torn leaf. It is a clear, jelly-like substance. Once prepared, it spoils within 2-3 days.

Aloe sap (sometimes called aloe juice or latex) is the brownish-red liquid which drips from between the outer leaf and the inner gel. If you collect and then heat this liquid, it will form a crystalline lump which is available, along with a dried, powdered form of the resin, at local Mid-Eastern herb shops. The Arabic word for dried aloe sap is *subr*.

IN THE KITCHEN

Having an aloe plant in or near the kitchen is convenient when it is time to harvest its thick leaves for cosmetic or medicinal purposes.

RESEARCH

Medical researchers at King Saud University in Riyadh have studied the effectiveness of aloe sap for treating blood sugar levels in diabetic patients. (see *Horm. Res.* 1986; 24(4): 288-94.)

Chinese scientists have reported significant antioxidant activity in aloe vera extracts. (Hu, Y., et al. 'Evaluation of Antioxidant Potential of Aloe vera (Aloe barbadensis Miller) Extracts.' J *Agric Food Chem.* 2003 Dec 17;51(26):7788-9.)

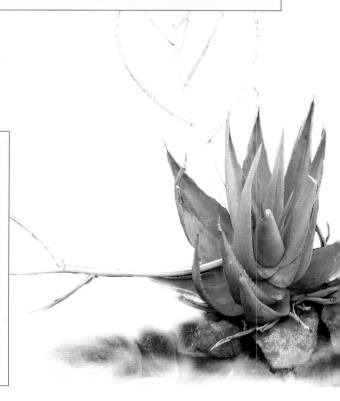

FAMILY REMEDIES ACROSS ARABIA

In the Arabian Peninsula, the dried sap of the aloe plant is a traditional remedy for diabetes. It is used to lower blood sugar levels and to treat slow-to-heal wounds. It is also a purgative to cleanse the stomach and intestines and is thus used internally to treat stomach complaints. Externally, the gel is used to promote the growth of beautiful hair.

Diabetes: Mix 100g shabba (*alum*), 100g myrrh, 200g arta, and 50g *subr* (dried aloe sap). Apply externally on cuts that won't heal due to diabetes. (Eastern KSA). ❧ Take a small piece of dried aloe sap with water twice a week to lower blood sugar. (Western KSA)

Caution: Repeated use can damage the liver, especially in the elderly (Western KSA).

Hair Treatment: For hair loss, use henna, garlic, castor oil, aloe and coconut (Central KSA) ❧ Put fresh aloe vera gel in the blender and mix well. Rub the hair with it to treat split ends, hair loss, and to strengthen the hair (Eastern KSA) ❧ Mix aloe vera gel with *sidr* and pomegranate peelings for beautiful healthy hair. (Eastern KSA)

Purgative: Soak a small piece of dried aloe sap in water for an hour. Drink. It cleanses the stomach and colon. (Western KSA)

DID YOU KNOW?

❧ The root of the Arabic word for aloe means 'patient, long-suffering, enduring'. In fact, the aloe plant has the capacity to endure hot, dry, desert conditions.

❧ In Saudi Arabia, *A. rubroviolaceae, A. tomentosa,* and *A. niebuhriana* have been reported growing in the Asir mountains, while *A. barbadensis* is widely cultivated.

❧ There are three main commercial varieties of aloe: Curaçao or Barbados aloe, named for its strong presence in the Caribbean (including *Aloe vera = A. barbadensis, A. officinalis* and *A. chinensis*); Socotrine aloe, from East Africa, Arabia and the island of Socotra (particularly *Aloe perryi*); Cape aloe, from southern Africa (including *Aloe ferox, A. spicata* and *A. Africana*).

❧ The aloe family consists of over 200 species, of which *Aloe vera* is considered the most effective healer.

❧ Some botanists consider *Aloe vera* to be a member of the large Lily Family (Liliaceae). But the modern trend has been to spin off monophyletic (common-ancestor) families from Liliaceae, and Aloeaceae is one of these.

❧ The ancient Egyptians probably employed aloe in the mummification process, and Queen Cleopatra is said to have used it to protect her skin from the sun.

❧ The medieval Arab philosopher and physician al-Kindi mentions aloe as an effective treatment for inflammatory pain, eye ulcers, melancholy and various medical problems. Aloe was also used in Persia as a purgative, and in Egypt as a detersive to clean the digestive system and detoxify the body.

ALUM

Arabic: *shabba, shabb*
Other English: Potassium Alum, Potash Alum

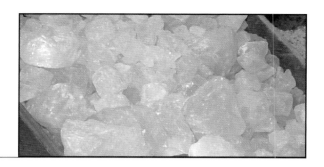

First-time visitors to Middle Eastern markets may be puzzled to see piles of stones displayed prominently among the herbs and spices. Shopkeepers offer porous black chunks of rock called *hajar* (stone), used as pumice. There is also white salt and black salt from Iran or India and *bukhoor jawi* (Javanese incense), collections of gray, black, and brownish-red stones from Java, which are burned for their fragrance. A mixture of many of these fragrant stones, crushed and blended together into one incense, is usually on-hand, ready to be burned. And, in almost all herb shops, there will be a crystal-white mineral, often imported from China, called *shabba*, and known in English as alum.

Alum is a compound of several metals, including aluminium. It is an astringent, widely used in the Middle East to control bleeding and to clean and heal wounds. Shabba powder is mixed with henna for skin decoration, and when applied to the underarms, it acts as a deodorant.

RESEARCH

A recent Turkish dentistry study found that daily use of a mouth rinse containing alum (hydrated aluminium potassium sulfate) was safe for children and significantly reduced levels of three types of oral Streptococcus in plaque and saliva. (Olmez, A., et al. 'Effect of an alum-containing mouthrinse in children for plaque and salivary levels of selected oral microflora.' *J Clin Pediatr Dent.* 1998 Summer; 22(4):335-40.)

At India's National Institute of Cholera & Enteric Diseases, potash alum was shown to work as an effective bactericide against a number of harmful intestinal microbes grown in vitro. (Dutta, S., et al. 'In vitro antimicrobial activity of potash alum.' *Indian J Med Res.* 1996 Jul;104:157-9.)

HOW TO USE

1. Use the stone whole.

2. Crush into small pieces.

3. Grind into a powder.

IN THE KITCHEN

Alum is not ingested, and is not used in cooking.

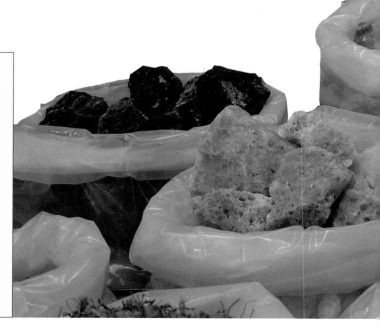

FAMILY REMEDIES ACROSS ARABIA

Bleeding: Apply *shabba* to stop bleeding. (Northern KSA) ❧ Use for infections on external cuts or wounds. (Northern KSA) ❧ For inflammations of mouth and cuts. (Eastern KSA)

Childbirth: Use *shabba* stone after delivery. (Northern KSA) ❧ As a suppository after childbirth to shrink the cells and tighten the vagina. (Eastern KSA) ❧ Grind to powder and mix 10g alum, 20g chamomile, and 10g salt. Combine this mixture with 5g gum Arabic and a little water to form a small tablet. Use this as a vaginal suppository after delivery. (Bahrain)

Cosmetics: Mix *shabba* stone powder with henna and lemon. It makes a dark colour to decorate the skin. (Northern KSA) ❧ Wash with *sidr* and *shabba*. (Eastern KSA) ❧ Grind the *shabba* stone and use as deodorant (Eastern KSA). ❧ Rub the powdered or stone form of alum under the arms as a deodorant. (Bahrain)

DID YOU KNOW?

☞ In ancient Babylon, physicians used alum in a mouthwash, as a styptic, as a pessary for menorrhagia, as a nasal douche, and as a treatment for itchy scabs, gonorrhea and purulent ophthalmia. Greek and then Arab medical authorities continued these practices, and went on to use alum for the treatment of leprosy, bad gums, pustules and ear trouble.

☞ The 9th-century encyclopedist Ibn Qutayba of Baghdad reports: 'In Yemen there is a mountain from which there drips water, and when it reaches the ground and dries [hardens], it changes and becomes [a kind of alum called] *shabb*. This is the well-known Yemenite *shabb*.' One commentator identifies this as *shabb zafar*, 'greasy alum,' which has a dirty, yellowish appearance and is also known as 'mountain butter.'

☞ Alums are valuable in paper manufacturing, textile dyeing, fireproofing, water purification, and in medicine as astringents, styptics and emetics.

☞ The Alum Mountain in Bulahdelah, Australia, is the only known above-ground outcrop of alum stone (alunite) in the world.

☞ Using *shabba* deodorant stones is considered safe and will not cause high levels of aluminium in your system. This is because potassium alum molecules have a negative ionic charge, and the aluminium is unable to pass through cell walls.

☞ Bauxite, the ore from which alum is drawn, can be purified and converted directly into alum. Bauxite is formed by the rapid weathering of granite rocks in warm, humid climates. Saudi Arabia has extensive bauxite deposits, and has announced plans to develop an aluminium industry.

ANISE

Pimpinella anisum
Apiaceae/Umbelliferae (Parsley) Family
Arabic: *anisun, yansun, yansoon*
Other English: Aniseed

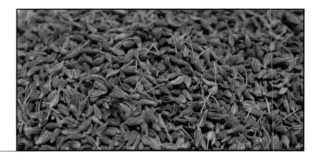

From cookies to colds, this tiny aromatic grey-brown seed – often called aniseed – serves families across the Arabian Peninsula. Saudi merchants import much of their aniseed from Syria and India. It is then made available at spice counters in supermarkets, outdoor weekend markets, and in local herbalist shops. Anise also grows in Egypt, Cyprus, Crete, and on the Eastern Mediterranean coast.

RECIPES	*Anise Cookies, p. 199* *Date Bars, p. 200*

HOW TO USE

1. For tea, simmer one teaspoon of aniseed in a cup of water for about ten minutes. Strain and drink.

2. Grind seeds to powder for use in baking.

3. Chew the seeds to freshen the mouth and aid digestion.

IN THE KITCHEN

Licorice-flavoured aniseeds provide subtle flavour to cookies and other sweets.

DID YOU KNOW?

⋐ Anise is sometimes confused with fennel (*Foeniculum vulgare*), particularly the Iranian varieties, which are quite similar in appearance and flavour.

⋐ The oil distilled from anise is what gives licorice candy its flavour.

⋐ Anise is a key ingredient of *supari*, the digestive spice mix served after a curry meal.

⋐ Arak, an aperitif distilled from grape juice and aniseed, is popular in the Middle East but is not available in Saudi Arabia due to its alcoholic content.

⋐ The Greek physician Galen (130-200 AD) prescribed aniseed as a diuretic, aphrodisiac and poison antidote.

RESEARCH

Anise has been known for thousands of years to function as an oestrogenic agent, increasing milk secretion, promoting menstruation, facilitating birth, etc. Research suggests that the pharmacologically active agents are polymers of anethole, the main constituent of anise seed essential oil. (Albert-Puleo, M. 'Fennel and anise as estrogenic agents.' *J. Ethnopharmacol.* 1980 Dec; 2(4): 337-44.)

Iranian researchers have noted that the essential oil of anise seed helps suppress convulsions in mice. (Pourgholami, M.H., et al. 'The fruit essential oil of Pimpinella anisum exerts anticonvulsant effects in mice.' *J. Ethnopharmacol.* 1999 Aug; 66(2): 211-5.)

FAMILY REMEDIES ACROSS ARABIA

Anise is a popular folk medicine, with a long tradition in Islamic pharmacology. It is used to treat general abdominal pain, colic, indigestion, menstrual cramping, coughs and headaches. It is also believed to clean the urinary system and prevent inflammations. Anise has aromatic, diaphoretic, relaxant, stimulant, tonic, carminative and stomachic properties.

Childbirth: To strengthen a mother following childbirth, feed her fenugreek, anise, black seeds and wheat. (Western KSA) ❧ Eat anise and dates. (Southern KSA)

Colic: Give the baby an infusion of a little myrrh and anise. Also, rub the baby's body at night with warm oil. (Central KSA) ❧ For a baby's stomachache, mix a drink of anise and honey in water. (Eastern KSA) ❧ To relieve colic, use anise and *sukr al-nabat*, a natural sugar similar in appearance to *shabba* (alum) but more translucent. (Eastern KSA) ❧ Boil equal quantities of anise, cumin and peppermint. Add crystalline sugar or honey. Then, add 7 drops of black seed oil and drink while warm. (Eastern KSA) ❧ For babies, use caraway, fenugreek, anise, water and sugar. (Eastern KSA)

Coughs: To relieve a cough, chew anise. (Eastern KSA ❧ Put a small amount of anise with the same amount of myrrh in a small bottle of water and let sit for one night. Before bedtime, drink two tablespoons (30 ml) of the liquid. (Central KSA) ❧ For upper respiratory tract infection, laryngitis or pharyngitis, boil 2-3 teaspoons *yansoon* in one cup of water and drink. (Eastern KSA)

Headaches: For headaches, combine a portion of powdered black seed with half the amount each of powdered clove and anise. Mix with a teaspoon of yogurt and eat. Then apply black seed oil to the painful area. (Eastern KSA)

Indigestion: For indigestion, boil and drink anise. (Central KSA)

Insomnia: For trouble sleeping, use nutmeg powder boiled like coffee and a small spoon of anise. Alternatively, drink anise and peppermint. (Central KSA)

Menstrual Cramps: For menstrual cramps, drink anise. (Southern KSA)

Stomach Pain: For general stomach pain, use cinnamon, cumin and anise. (Southern KSA) ❧ For a stomachache, use anise. Boil it and drink just like tea. It can be sweetened with sugar. (Western KSA)

Stress: To relax, drink anise and chamomile tea. (Central KSA)

Toothache: Add aniseed to tea to cure mild colds and dull toothaches. (UAE)

ARAK

Salvadora persica L.
Salvadoraceae Family
Arabic: *arak, rak, miswak, siwak*
Other English: Toothbrush Tree, Mustard
Tree, Saltbush

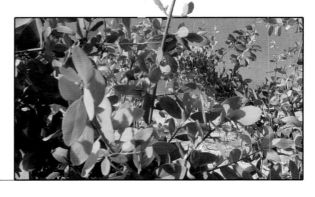

Have you ever wondered how people cleaned their teeth before the invention of the toothbrush? One answer is the *miswak*. A *miswak* (plural: *masawik*) is a fibrous stick prepared from the root of the arak tree. It has antiseptic and astringent properties which help clean and protect the teeth and gums. A high-quality miswak has a strong pungent smell. It is pale yellow or cream in colour. It is moist and flexible.

The Prophet Muhammad recommended the *miswak* to his followers. He used it to sweeten his breath during fasting and advised its use prior to prayer. This practice is still popular in Arabia today.

The arak is a short evergreen tree that grows in sandy and arid areas of the Middle East and Africa. Sheep and goats like to nibble its leaves.

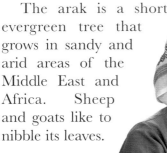

HOW TO USE

Soak the root in water for a few hours to soften the natural fibres. Scrape off $1/4$ to $1/2$ inch of bark from the tip and gently chew until fibres have separated and the root becomes brush-like. Clean the teeth by rubbing the *miswak* up and down and sideways as you would a conventional plastic toothbrush. When the fibres become overused, simply cut off the tip of the *miswak*, scrape off more bark, and continue to use as before.

IN THE KITCHEN

To retain freshness, keep *miswak* in the refrigerator or soak in water.

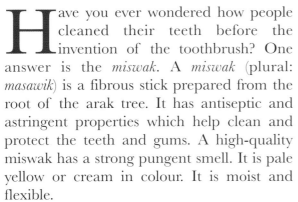

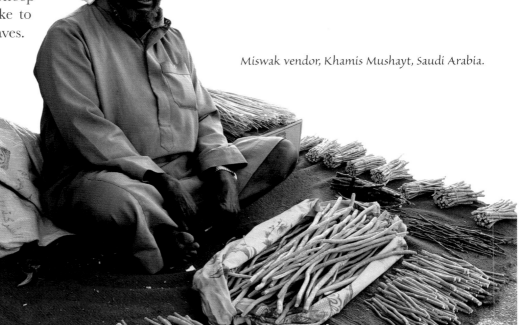

Miswak vendor, Khamis Mushayt, Saudi Arabia.

FAMILY REMEDIES ACROSS ARABIA

Miswak is used by Bedouin, townsfolk and city dwellers to clean and protect teeth and gums.

DID YOU KNOW?

❧ *Miswak* (sometimes called *siwak*) is sold by street vendors in the Middle East, oftentimes outside mosques. It is also available pre-packaged in pharmacies and supermarkets.

❧ Although *miswak* is described as 'pleasantly bitter', it is known to leave your breath sweeter. It also removes plaque from the teeth.

❧ Arak roots contain triclosan, an effective antibacterial used in modern toothpastes. Other ingredients include fluoride, vitamin C, alkaloids and small amounts of tannins and flavenoids.

❧ A herbal toothpaste with pure *miswak* extract (made by a hygiene products company in India) is currently marketed in Saudi Arabia and other countries of the region.

❧ Other natural toothbrush sources, when arak is not available, include the Peelo tree, the Olive tree, the Bitam tree, the Walnut tree, the Neem tree, or any bitter tree that is not harmful or poisonous in any way!

❧ A well-known grove of these medicinal trees grew until the 1950s at a location north of Dhahran near the Gulf coast village of Rakah (which itself means 'Toothbrush Tree'), the birthplace of Ali I. Al-Naimi, Saudi Minister of Petroleum and Mineral Resources.

❧ South Arabian historian al-Hamdani (d. 945) recorded that the ancient city of Ma'rib in Yemen, capital of the Kingdom of Saba or Sheba, 'has more arak trees than any other city.' He adds: 'The ring-doves which swarm the arak trees are beyond description.'

RESEARCH

A recent survey of Saudi Bedouins conducted by the King Saud University College of Dentistry found that 25 per cent of them used only *miswak* for oral hygiene while 30 per cent used both *miswak* and toothbrush. (Almas, K., et al. 'Oral hygiene, dietary pattern and smoking habits of Bedouin (nomadic Arabs) population in Saudi Arabia.' *Odontostomatol Trop.* 2003 Sep; 26 (103): 19-23.)

A decoction of *Salvadora persica* root has been shown to have a significant protective effect against ulcers induced in rats. (Monforte, M.T. 'Antiulcer Activity'. *Pharmaceutical Biology*, 2001, Vol.39, No.4, pp. 289-92.)

ARTA

Calligonum polygonoides or *C. comosum*
Polygonaceae (Rhubarb) Family
Arabic: *arta* (North Arabia), *abal* (Bahrain &
    Saudi Arabia)

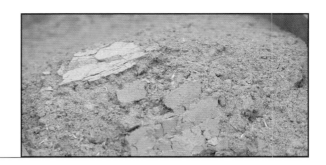

A young Bedouin astride his camel finds arta growing on the sand dunes near his encampment. He notices sizeable bushes – a metre or more in height – with very small needle-like leaves and long red roots stabilizing the surrounding sand into large mounds. The bushes have an appealing fragrance. In the early springtime months of March and April, he sees the bright red fruits he knows as *nathara*. He carefully dismounts and approaches arta with anticipation. His mother and grandmother, who use arta for practical and medicinal purposes, will be very happy to receive this desert bounty.

To the Bedouin, arta is not simply another desert plant growing on the dunes of Central and Eastern Saudi Arabia. Its branches make excellent firewood. Its leaves and twigs generate cash flow when sold in the local market. Its fruit is edible and used as a mouth freshener.

HOW TO USE

Dry the leaves and fine twigs and then grind into powder.

IN THE KITCHEN

Before the conveniences of modern piping and refrigeration, leather bags were made to store and carry water and milk. Arta was used to tan the insides of these leather bags prior to use. Saudi Bedouins of the Dahna desert sometimes still use arta for this purpose. Those in the 'Ain Dar area of Eastern Saudi Arabia use a mixture of ground arta leaves and honey to coat the inside of goatskin bags to add flavour to camel's milk.

Abu Mansur, a respected Persian physician of the 10th century, reported that milk skins were tanned with arta leaves and the flavour of the milk improved in them. Nowadays, the red roots of arta are sometimes still used for tanning skins.

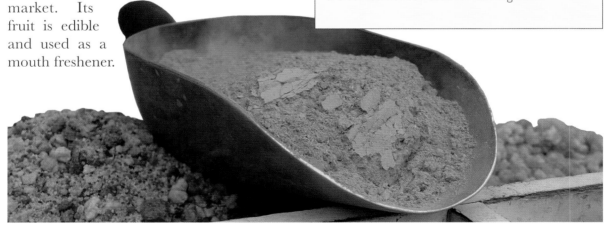

RESEARCH

Arta extract has been shown to have a significant anti-inflammatory effect in laboratory rats. It also inhibits acute gastric ulcers in rats. (Liu, X.M., et al. 'Anti-inflammatory and anti-ulcer activity of *Calligonum comosum* in rats.' *Fitoterapia*, 2001, 72:487-91.)

Other research on rats has shown arta to have positive cardiovascular effects. (Radhakrishnan, R., et al. 'Cardiovascular effects of *Calligonum comosum* extract in rat.' J *Pharm Pharmacol.* 1999, 51 (Suppl):119.)

FAMILY REMEDIES ACROSS ARABIA

Childbirth: (*Treatments for strengthening or cleansing mothers are generally followed during the 40 days after childbirth.*) Boil arta twigs with pomegranate peelings and wash a mother's sore areas with the liquid. Alternatively, mix three spoons of powdered arta with 1.5 litres of water. Add natural salt if desired, and wash a mother's sore areas with the liquid. (KSA) ⤛ To cleanse a mother following childbirth, use vaginal suppositories formed with powdered arta, natural salt, myrrh and *maqalah*, a substance from Iran. (Eastern KSA)

Diabetes: For wounds that refuse to heal due to diabetes, grind and mix the following: 4 cups arta, 2 cups myrrh, 1 cup white *shabba* (alum), and 1 cup black seed (*Nigella sativa*). Place the mixture on/in the wound and cover with a bandage. Replace regularly. Within a week the wound will heal. It helps prevent gangrene. (Eastern KSA) ⤛ Use 100g *shabba*, 100g myrrh, 200g arta, and 50g *subr* (dried aloe sap). Apply externally on cuts that won't heal due to diabetes. (Eastern KSA)

Flatulence (Intestinal Gas): To dissipate gas formed by drinking milk or buttermilk, add $^1/_2$ teaspoon of arta powder to the milk or else, separately, mix $^1/_2$ teaspoon arta powder with a glass of water and drink. (KSA)

Skin Ailments: Use powdered *abal* leaves in a balm to treat skin ailments. (Bahrain)

Stomach Ulcers: To cure a stomach ulcer, dry grated pomegranate peelings and arta twigs. Grind with some crystallized sugar (*sukkar nabat*), in a mortar and pestle. Take a spoonful of the mixture, blended in milk, every morning and the ulcer will vanish in time (Eastern KSA). Take a small spoonful of arta powder with milk and honey every morning for 20 days. (KSA)

DID YOU KNOW?

⤛ In Eastern Saudi Arabia, women at the Hofuf Thursday market sell arta in fine twig and powdered form.

⤛ Arta grows abundantly in the deserts of Saudi Arabia. As a precautionary measure, however, Saudi Arabia has recently banned local harvesting to preserve this plant.

⤛ An extinct volcano in the Kingdom's Western Province, southeast of Tabuk, is named Umm Arta (Mother of Arta). Explorer Alois Musil, visiting the surrounding area in 1910, found arta growing in many places, on sand dunes and in flat plains. His party's camels were always happy to graze on the plants.

⤛ Bedouins in the UAE used the young shoots as a vegetable and the red fruits as a spice.

⤛ Along the main highways of the UAE, fences have been erected to protect camels and goats from speeding cars. As well as protecting animals, these fences provide a ten-metre-wide strip free from animal grazing. Arta thrives in this animal-free zone. Elsewhere it is under threat of local extinction due to intense grazing.

⤛ The disappearance of arta impacts several species of nocturnal moths, whose larvae feed on it. The loss of their food source could have far-reaching effects on desert flora throughout the region.

⤛ US soldiers who have served in the Middle East recommend eating arta flowers when stranded in the desert and in survival mode.

ARUGULA

Eruca sativa
Brassicaceae/Cruciferae (Cabbage) Family
Arabic: *jarjeer, jirjir*
Other English: Rocket, Roquette

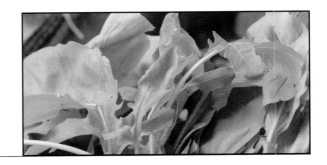

An old Egyptian saying observes that if people knew what was in *jarjeer*, they would plant it under the bed. The ancient Egyptians and Romans regarded the oil of *Eruca sativa* as an aphrodisiac. The plant's reputation survives to this day in the Middle East and other regions.

In Saudi Arabia, where arugula is eaten as a vegetable, it is said to prevent disease and generally strengthen health. The plant has an array of other medicinal uses. For example, its juice is used to treat cuts and burns and even to remove freckles.

Jarjeer is sometimes called *baqla Aisha* (Aisha's vegetable) after a wife of the Prophet Muhammad.

HOW TO USE

1. Wash fresh leaves and add them to salads or other recipes.

2. Squeeze the leaves to extract juice for various medicinal uses.

3. Use *jarjeer* seeds as a spice.

IN THE KITCHEN

Jarjeer is served with *kuba* (an Arabic meat dish). It is used to decorate or garnish food and as a salad green. *Jarjeer* leaves have a slight peppery flavour and are delicious served with onions and tomatoes. In eastern Saudi Arabia, it is popular with fish dishes.

Jarjeer is valued for its iron content.

RECIPE	Arugula and Pomegranate Salad, p.185

DID YOU KNOW?

🐛 Sometimes *jarjeer* is erroneously identified as another member of the cabbage family, watercress (*Nasturtium officinale*). Like *Eruca sativa*, watercress has a fresh, clean peppery taste – though a bit milder than arugula.

🐛 In medieval times, Arab alchemist Jabir ibn Hayyan (known as Geber to the Europeans) used arugula in a plaster to draw out poisons, including scorpion venom.

🐛 Al-Kindi, the 9th-century Arab philosopher and physician, names arugula seed in a complex 'black remedy' for insanity. The medicine includes

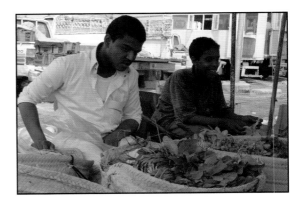

Vegetable market, al-Hasa, Saudi Arabia.

some 37 ingredients (among them euphorbium and opium!). Al-Kindi calls it 'useful for attacks of madness, epilepsy, weakness, all cold ailments and black bile.'

🐛 The Jewish Mishna and Talmud mention use of *jarjeer* in the Holy Land during the Hellenistic period as a treatment for eye infections, an aphrodisiac, a deodorant, a protection against dog bites and a digestive aid.

FAMILY REMEDIES ACROSS ARABIA

Blood Cleanser: When added to your food, it makes your blood clean. (Northern KSA) ❧ *Jarjeer* aids digestion and removes impurities from the blood. (Eastern KSA)

Burns: Use *jarjeer* ointment for old burns, prepared as follows: take a quantity of *jarjeer* with a medium onion and a quantity of strawberry leaves and cook. Strain the mixture while hot through a piece of gauze and use to treat skin infections with pus. (Eastern KSA)

Constipation: Useful for treating constipation and it stimulates the appetite. (Central KSA)

Diarrhoea: Use *jarjeer* juice mixed with1 tablespoon powdered black seed. Drink a cup of the mixture 3 times a day until diarrhoea ends on the second day. Then stop to avoid constipation. (Eastern KSA)

Fatigue: We use *jarjeer* because it contains iron to strengthen the blood and give it energy. (KSA)

Fevers: Eat the leaves to treat fever. (Eastern KSA)

Hair Loss: Rocket is good – we put its water or its oil in our hair to prevent hair loss. (Central KSA) ❧ It removes freckles and loss of pigment resulting in white skin and is used to treat hair loss. Mix 150g of *jarjeer* juice with 50g of vinegar and apply to scalp every day for a month. (Eastern KSA) ❧ Apply castor oil, henna and *jarjeer* oil. (Northern KSA) ❧ Garlic, lemon and *jarjeer*. (Central KSA) ❧ Sesame oil, garlic, jarjeer, jarjeer oil and black seed oil. (Southern KSA) ❧ For hair loss, use henna, egg, *sidr*, olive oil, aloe vera, *jarjeer* juice, parsley and garlic. (Eastern KSA ❧ Use powdered black seed in *jarjeer* juice with a tablespoon of diluted vinegar and one *finjan* olive oil and rub the head in the evening before bedtime. Then wash with warm water and shampoo every day. (Eastern KSA) ❧ Use a mix of oils, including almond and sesame, with onion juice and garlic. *Jarjeer* oil and henna are put on hair with hibiscus. (Eastern KSA) ❧ *Jarjeer* is good for the hair, especially its oil. When eaten, it's good for the blood. (UAE) ❧ We generally use *jarjeer* in salads; it is good for the blood, skin and hair. *Jarjeer* oil nourishes and strengthens hair. (Bahrain and UAE)

Indigestion: First blend and squeeze the leaves to extract the juice. Give the sick person 1 tablespoon three times a day, but don't drink *jarjeer* juice a lot because it may cause digestive problems. (Eastern KSA) ❧ Use honey, *jarjeer*, *karrath* (leeks), dates and cress. Mix dates and cress with a little amount of butter and eat it while warm – it's very nourishing. (Central KSA)

Sexual Vigour: Many women believe that eating *jarjeer* is excellent for their sexual relationship (Northern KSA) ❧ It stimulates sexual desire and strengthens the blood. It is eaten as a salad. (Eastern KSA)

RESEARCH

Arugula seed oil has antioxidant properties. A recent Egyptian university study found that the oil relieves oxidative stress associated with diabetes mellitus in rats. (El-Missiry, M.A., and A.M. El Gindy. 'Amelioration of alloxan induced diabetes mellitus and oxidative stress in rats by oil of *Eruca sativa* seeds.' *Ann Nutr Metab*. 2000; 44(3): 97-100.)

ASAFOETIDA

Ferula assa-foetida or F. asafoetida
Apiaceae/Umbelliferae (Parsley) Family
Arabic: *haltita, hiltit*
Other English: Asafetida, Giant Fennel,
   Devil's Dung, Stinking Gum, Food of the
   Gods

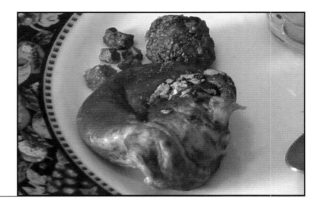

When the doorbell rang, young Khalid knew that his grandmother had arrived with that infamous family remedy of hers: the foul-smelling gum resin of the asafoetida plant. His mind raced to find an excuse, any excuse, to avoid taking it. He doubted that the effort it took to swallow the bitter substance was worth the cure. Yet he knew his grandmother would be firm. Her refrain was always the same, and today was no different:

'You know, Khalid, asafoetida has been used for ages as an effective medicine in the Arab world. It works mainly to improve digestion, but it's also a pain-reliever, a cough medicine and a blood thinner. We'll use it to treat your upset stomach.'

Khalid had no choice but to agree ... and sure enough, he soon felt better.

In Saudi Arabia today, families still turn to asafoetida as a 'last resort' treatment for coughs, colds, fevers and stomach discomfort. It is not the most popular home remedy – parents coach their children to hold their noses and swallow quickly to tolerate the strong smell and bitter taste.

HOW TO USE

1. Dissolve in water and drink.

2. Grind or crush the lump resin into powder or dissolve it in liquid and use sparingly as a cooking spice.

IN THE KITCHEN

Despite its sulfurous smell, asafoetida, when cooked, imparts a surprisingly pleasant flavour to many foods. In Indian cuisine, it is a substitute for onion or garlic. Use in small amounts. The powdered form is milder than the resin, because it is normally blended with rice flour. The resin should be fried in hot oil before using. A pea-sized quantity is enough to flavor a large pot of lentils or vegetables. Store asafoetida in an air-tight container.

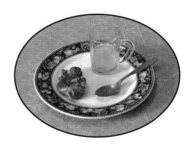

RESEARCH

U.S. Department of Agriculture research finds that asafetida has antifungal properties, controlling both the growth and aflatoxin production of the fungus *Aspergillus flavus*. (Takeoka, Gary R. 'Volatile Constituents of Asafoetida.' TEKTRAN (Agricultural Research Service), Jan. 14, 2000.)

In Nepal, asafetida is used in very small amounts for a number of traditional medicinal purposes. (Eigner, D., and D. Scholz. '*Ferula asa-foetida* and *Curcuma longa* in traditional medical treatment and diet in Nepal.' *J Ethnopharmacol* 1999 Oct; 67(1):1-6.)

FAMILY REMEDIES ACROSS ARABIA

Asafoetida is available in Middle Eastern herb shops and can be purchased in lump resin or powdered form.

Coughs, Colds, Stomach Discomfort and Fever: Put a small piece, half an inch in diameter, in a small glass container and add half a cup water. Let it sit in the refrigerator until needed. It lasts for up to a month. For children, one teaspoon will normally bring a fever down and relieve stomach upset within a short time. It can be repeated the next day if necessary. (Central KSA)

Sore Throats: Soak myrrh and asafoetida in water. Strain and drink. (Central and Northern KSA)

Toothache: If you have a painful tooth cavity, insert a small piece of asafoetida in the cavity to relieve the pain. (Socotra, Yemen)

DID YOU KNOW?

🐛 Asafoetida is native to Iran and western Afghanistan.

🐛 Modern herbalists regard asafoetida as a sedative, antispasmodic and circulatory agent. It is also known to relieve intestinal and stomach upsets.

🐛 John Heinerman, in his book *Miracle Healing Herbs*, recommends putting ⅛ teaspoon crumbled dried asafoetida in a cup of hot water and letting it simmer for 15 minutes before drinking. This suggestion is based on the folk medicine of Kazakhstan. People who have tried it report positive effects against tension headaches.

🐛 Asafoetida is much used in the Ayurvedic tradition and is also popular in Indian vegetarian cooking.

🐛 Al-Kindi, an Arab physician of the 9th century AD, used asafoetida to counter phlegm and treat sore throat, tooth pain, rheumatism and nervous conditions, and also as an aphrodisiac.

🐛 Alexander the Great is credited with bringing asafoetida back to the west in the 4th century BC, after his expeditions into the Persian Empire (modern Afghanistan).

🐛 The British explorer Charles Doughty, who travelled throughout Arabia in the mid-19th century, called asafoetida 'a drug which the Arabs have in sovereign estimation.'

🐛 Asafoetida is an ingredient in some Worcestershire sauce recipes.

🐛 Asafoetida gets its name from the Persian *aza*, for mastic or resin, and the Latin *foetidus*, for stinking.

Khalid Al-Dhubaib, al-Khobar, Saudi Arabia, dutifully takes asafoetida.

BANANA

Musa sapientum
Musaceae (Banana) Family
Arabic: *mauz*

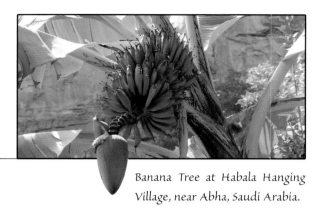

Banana Tree at Habala Hanging Village, near Abha, Saudi Arabia.

The banana plant is the world's largest herb. It is often mistaken for a tree, but does not have a woody trunk or boughs. It springs from an underground rhizome to form a false trunk 3-6 metres high and is crowned with a rosette of 10-20 beautiful, oblong-shaped banana leaves.

History credits Arab traders with giving the banana its popular name. Although there are several hundred varieties which differ in taste, colour, form, and size, Arab traders noted that bananas growing in Africa and Asia were small, about the size of a man's finger, and so called them *banan*, which means 'fingertips' in Arabic. 'Banana' is the singular form.

Bananas are rich in potassium, riboflavin, niacin and dietary fibre. They also contain vitamins A and C and some calcium and iron. Bananas are a quick source of energy.

HOW TO USE

Banana plants are extremely versatile. In banana-producing countries, vegetables and spices are sometimes wrapped in banana leaves and then steamed. Banana leaves are used as serving plates, as table cloths, and as barriers between a wood fire and a pot. They are even used for thatching roofs and making rope.

Bananas can be eaten fresh or dried. The dried fruit can be ground into a nutritious banana flour.

IN THE KITCHEN

A very old and traditional breakfast in Mecca is omelette with banana. *Masoub*, also featuring the banana, is currently a popular breakfast dish in Saudi Arabia's Western Province. *Kanafa* (an Arab pastry of shredded wheat or shredded filo) with banana is a delicious dessert.

RECIPES	Omelette with Banana, p. 182	Masoub, p. 182

DID YOU KNOW?

🐘 Hundreds of banana varieties thrive in the tropics. Bananas grow in Egypt, Yemen, Oman and other Arab countries. In the Nile River, near Luxor, Egypt, local boats sail to Gazirat al-Mauz (Banana Island), where visitors can sample fruits from a large banana orchard.

🐘 The banana has been cultivated in India for at least 4,000 years. Bananas are widely used in Indian folk medicine for the treatment of diabetes mellitus.

🐘 The celebrated Iraqi-born scientist Abdul Latif al-Baghdadi (1162-1231 AD), who taught medicine at Mosul, Cairo and Damascus, says the banana 'is aphrodisiac and diuretic and it gives flatulence.' The intestinal gas from bananas 'has an agreeable smell' unlike other digestive gases, he asserts.

🐘 A classic American dessert, the banana split, became popular in the 1920s. It consists of a banana split lengthwise in half and covered with three scoops of ice cream with chocolate and strawberry syrup, chopped nuts, and a maraschino cherry on top.

FAMILY REMEDIES ACROSS ARABIA

In our 2002 survey of families from the five regions of Saudi Arabia, the banana surfaced as a prominent remedy.

Childbirth: Sweet gruel – a traditional hot cereal that includes dates, banana and honey – is a remedy to help strengthen a mother after childbirth. (Central KSA)

Diarrhoea: Take cornstarch mixed in water; yoghurt; tea leaves; mashed potatoes; or bananas. (Bahrain) ๑ Take rice water and banana. (Southern KSA) ๑ Eat banana and *laban* or banana, yoghurt and cornstarch. (Western KSA) ๑ Take yoghurt, banana, white rice, 7-Up (lemon-lime soft drink) and green lemon. (Central KSA)

Healthy Skin: In the past, women used banana paste as a mask to moisten skin. (Eastern KSA)

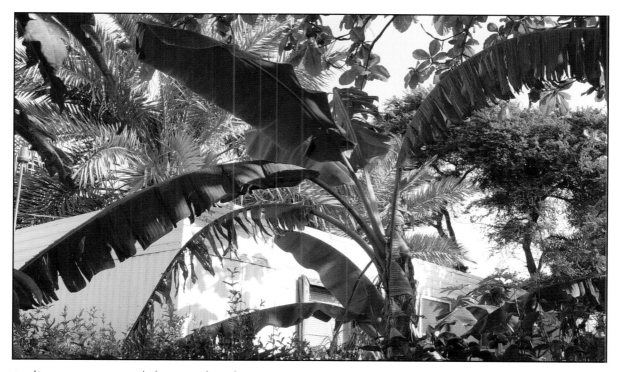

Saudi Aramco Nursery, Dhahran, Saudi Arabia.

RESEARCH

Doctors at Pennsylvania Hospital in Philadelphia found that banana flakes can be used as a safe, cost-effective treatment for diarrhoea in critically ill tube-fed patients. (Emery, E.A. 'Banana flakes control diarrhea in enterally fed patients.' *Nutr Clin Pract* 1997 Apr;12(2):72-5.)

Banana flower extract has been shown to lower blood sugar levels in diabetic rats. (Pari, L. et al. 'Antihyperglycaemic activity of *Musa sapientum* flowers: effect on lipid peroxidation in alloxan diabetic rats.' *Phytother Res* 2000 Mar;14(2):136-8.)

BASIL, SWEET

Ocimum basilicum
Lamiaceae (Mint) Family
Arabic: *rayhan, reehan, mashmum*

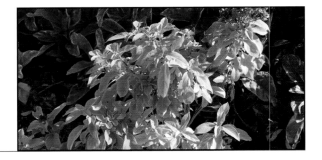

A 40-year-old woman from the Najd, the Saudi heartland, was asked what remedies her mother or grandmother used that are not employed today. The memories came flooding back, and before long she was enthusiastically revealing some of the traditional uses of basil in central Saudi Arabia:

'Yes, there is basil,' she said with a smile. 'When you smell it you feel happy, and smelling it prevents diseases. And when you crush its leaves and mix them with vinegar and put [the mixture] on your head, it stops nosebleeds. When you put it on pimples or skin infections that produce pus in the hands and feet, it cures them. When you rub the body with basil, it prevents sweating, dries perspiration and removes odours from underarms. And when you sit on the mixture [of crushed leaves], it removes abscesses from the bottom and uterus.'

Nowadays, fragrant basil-leaf necklaces are sold at Thursday morning markets in many parts of Arabia. These necklaces have traditionally been worn at wedding parties. One Saudi Aramco employee reports that when work requires long absences from family, wives in al-Hasa spread basil on the bed and around the house as a provocative welcome-home gesture for their husbands. In al-Hasa and Qatif, basil is grown year-round.

HOW TO USE

1. Place basil leaves in hair, clothing and houses for the lovely scent they give off.

2. Crush the dried leaves for various medicinal uses.

3. Rinse fresh leaves prior to use in the kitchen.

IN THE KITCHEN

Basil has many culinary uses in the Peninsula.

Amina Al-Ghamdi of al-Baha in southern Saudi Arabia says the women of her hometown often put about four basil leaves in a newly purchased carton of buttermilk (*laban*), to give it a special flavour when it's drunk the following day. However, she cautions that the buttermilk should be consumed within three days 'or the flavour will be stronger than it should be.'

Mahdi Al-Jamed of Qatif, in eastern Saudi Arabia, notes that basil is popular with tomatoes: 'A basil and tomato salad is fantastic. You can also add basil leaves to a regular salad.'

Wajeeha Huwaider of al-Hasa observes that some people in her area eat basil 'with anything that comes with bread, usually with dry food like kabab or white cheese. They learned that from the Iraqis, who eat it with just about any kind of food. So actually the Hasawi people [Shiites] with ties to Iraq eat *reehan*.'

RESEARCH

Antioxidant activity (rosmarinic acid) has been detected in extracts of sweet basil by Japanese and Sri Lankan researchers. (Jayasinghe, C., et al. 'Phenolics Composition and Antioxidant Activity of Sweet Basil (*Ocimum basilicum* L.).' *J Agric Food Chem.* 2003 Jul 16; 51(15): 4442-9.) Antimicrobial and antifungal properties have also been observed in recent studies.

FAMILY REMEDIES ACROSS ARABIA

Ant Bites: Rub the squeezed juice of basil leaves on the bite to reduce itching and inflammation. (Southern KSA)

Colds or Coughs: Take a warm drink of boiled basil with peppermint and lemon juice sweetened with crystalline sugar 2-3 times a day. (Eastern KSA).

Cuts: To speed healing, rub basil leaves on wounds and squeeze the juice of basil leaves over the wounds. (Eastern KSA)

Indigestion: Take a dried herb mixture of chamomile, green tea, peppermint and basil. (Southern KSA) ᐂ Eat soaked peppermint and basil. (Eastern KSA)

Insomnia: For trouble sleeping, eat peppermint and basil. (Southern KSA)

Stress: For relaxation, drink basil tea and/or soak your feet in basil and warm water. (Eastern KSA)

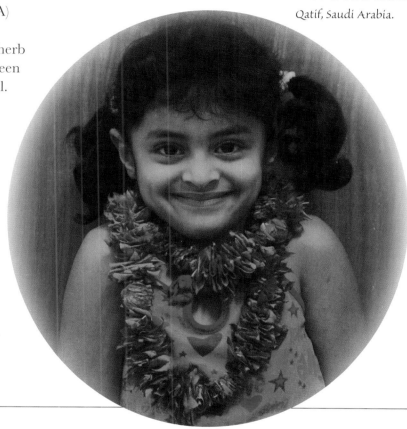

Samar Mahdi Al-Jamed wears a basil necklace, Qatif, Saudi Arabia.

DID YOU KNOW?

ᐂ In ancient times, the Greek physician Dioscorides considered basil to be a remedy for flatulence, bad eyesight, melancholy and the pain of a scorpion bite.

ᐂ In Iran, basil seeds are traditionally prescribed in a cold infusion for influenza.

ᐂ Culpeper, the 17th-century English herbalist, stated with regard to basil: 'Being applied to the place bitten by venomous beasts, or stung by a wasp or hornet, it speedily draws the poison to it.'

ᐂ Hindus are buried with a basil leaf on the breast. It is considered a passport to paradise.

ᐂ In Ayurvedic medicine, basil is known as *tulsi*.

ᐂ Basil is an important component of Italian food and the main ingredient in pesto.

BLACK SEED

Nigella sativa
Ranunculaceae (Buttercup) Family
Arabic: *habba souda, habbat al-barakah*
Other English: Fennel Flower, Black Cumin

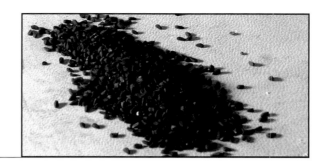

Nigella sativa is native to the Mediterranean and is grown throughout the Middle East and parts of Asia. It is cultivated for its seeds, which are known as the 'seeds of blessing.' For the Arabs, black seed is not only a food but also a valued traditional medicine that has long been used to treat such ailments as asthma, flatulence, polio, kidney stones, abdominal pain, etc. It has served as an important health and beauty aid for thousands of years.

According to tradition, the Prophet Muhammad described black seed as a cure for every disease except death! The great physician Ibn Sina (980-1037), better known as Avicenna, stated that black seed works as an expectorant, stimulates the body's energy and helps overcome fatigue and dispiritedness. Among the ancient Greeks, the physician Dioscorides prescribed black seed for nasal congestion, headaches, toothaches and intestinal parasites. Hippocrates found *Nigella sativa* useful in treating various hepatic and digestive disorders.

Black seed oil is very popular in Saudi Arabia and other Gulf countries and is sold in bottles for hair and skin care as well as for general health purposes. The seed is also used in various bread recipes originating in Turkey, Iran and India, and as a flavouring in a number of vegetable dishes.

HOW TO USE

1. Eat black seeds plain.

2. Eat a teaspoon of black seed mixed with honey.

3. Boil black seed with water. Strain and drink.

4. Heat black seed and warm milk until it just begins to boil. Remove from heat. Cool, then drink.

5. Grind black seed and swallow it with water or milk.

6. Sprinkle on bread and pastries before baking.

7. Burn black seed with *bukhoor* (incense) for a pleasant scent.

IN THE KITCHEN

Black seed is aromatic with a slight peppery flavour. It is one of the distinctive flavours of Arabic pastries. It is often sprinkled on breads and cheese. It is heated with milk for flavour. It is eaten ground with honey or with cakes and pastries.

RECIPES

Cheese Pie, p. 191
Qursan, p. 194
Saudi Sambusa, p. 193

Fried Dough Chips, p. 200
Aish Bi Laham, p. 195

FAMILY REMEDIES ACROSS ARABIA

In Arabia, black seed remains a traditional remedy for asthma, coughs, stomachache, abdominal pain, colic, general fatigue, rheumatism, mouth and larynx diseases, skin diseases and cancer. It is also believed to strengthen a mother after childbirth, stimulate menstruation, urination and liver functions, aid digestion, dissolve kidney stones, and increase intelligence. Black seed is used to beautify skin, nourish hair and stimulate hair growth.

Acne: Black seeds are ground and mixed with honey to get rid of acne and to clear facial skin. (Bahrain)

Asthma: To treat asthma, take black seed with honey. (Northern KSA)

Bones: Black seed is used with henna for the hair and with honey for the bones. (Southern KSA)

Childbirth: Drink milk with sweetened sesame and crystalline sugar or black seed boiled with honey or boiled chamomile (Eastern KSA). ᕗ During labour, drink milk with a tablespoon of ground black seeds (Eastern KSA). ᕗ Take black seed right after delivery. (Northern KSA)

Colds: Grind black seed and wrap it in a cloth to sniff. (Central KSA)

Colic: Boil anise, cumin and peppermint in equal quantities. Add some crystalline sugar or honey, then add 7 drops of black seed oil and drink while hot. (Eastern KSA)

(continued overleaf)

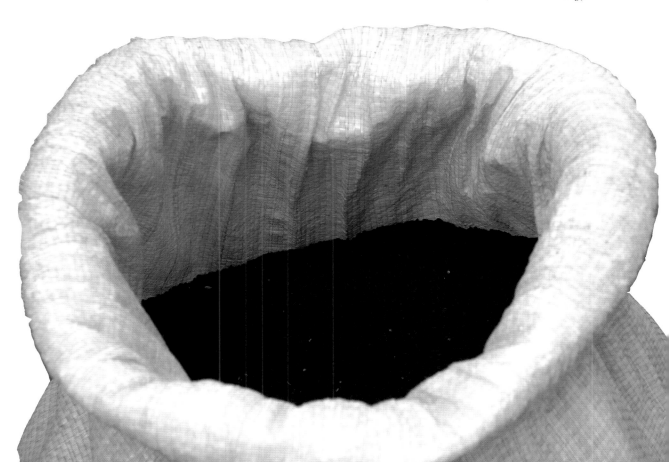

FAMILY REMEDIES ACROSS ARABIA (*cont.*)

Coughs: Mix ground black seed with honey and take a full spoon every morning for relief from coughs and to strengthen the body. (Northern KSA) ✿ For coughs or colds, take ginger, honey and black seed. Rub the chest with olive oil and a little Vicks. (Central KSA)

Diabetes: Mix 1 tablespoon of myrrh, 1 cup of cress, $^1/_2$ cup of black seed, $^1/_2$ cup of ground pomegranate, 1 cup of dried ground cabbage root, and a small spoon of cumin seeds with yogurt (to make it easier to eat). Eat on an empty stomach. (Eastern KSA)

Hair Loss: Use powdered black seed in *jarjeer* [arugula] juice with a tablespoon of diluted vinegar and a *finjan* of olive oil. Rub the head with this mixture every evening before bed. Wash hair in the morning with warm water and shampoo. Also, rub the scalp with onion juice before sleeping and wash in the morning with warm water and repeat until hair loss stops. (Eastern KSA). ✿ Try garlic, *jarjeer* oil, sesame oil and black seed oil. (Southern KSA)

Heart Trouble: Take a teaspoon of black seed in water every morning. (Western KSA)

Kidney Stones: Black seed has many benefits. One is that when ground and mixed with honey and drunk with hot water it melts the stones in kidneys and stimulates menstruation and urination. (Central KSA)

Nausea: Boil cloves with black seeds and drink without sweeteners three times a day (you may not need third dose). This is good for vomiting and nausea. (Eastern KSA)

Rheumatism: To treat rheumatism and pain in the joints, add black seed to olive oil and fennel. (Northern KSA)

Stomachache: Black seed is used with honey, cress, and fenugreek. All together are used as a medication for stomachaches and after giving birth. It's taken twice a day. (Eastern KSA) ✿ Use black seed in food for women right after delivery and as seed (swallow without cooking) for stomach pain. (Central KSA) ✿ Boil black seeds [in water], sweeten and drink. This is used as a diuretic and is also good for headaches and stomachaches. (Bahrain) ✿ Black seed with honey is good for stomach problems. (UAE)

Toothache, Tonsil and Larynx Pain: I use black seed for toothache, tonsil and larynx pain, by boiling it and using it as a gargle. Also, swallow a spoonful of black seed with warm water on an empty stomach every day. Rub the larynx and the gums with black seed oil. (Eastern KSA)

RESEARCH

Research: Black seed has long been known as a bronchodilator, providing relief for breathing problems. (El-Dakhakhny, M. 'Egyptian *Nigella sativa.' Arzneimittel-Forsch.* 15. 1227-29.)

Various tests of *Nigella sativa* oil on animals have shown significant antioxidant effects. One review of the literature concluded: 'On the basis of these results, it has been suggested that a nutritional supplement of the black seed extract may offer better protection to the human body against oxidative damage than supplementation with synthetic antioxidants.' (Khan, M.A. 'Chemical composition and medicinal properties of *Nigella sativa* Linn.' *Inflammopharmacology,* Vol. 7, No. 1, pp. 15-35 (1999).)

Black seed extract assists the human immune system by increasing the number and activity of immune competent cells. (Medenica, R., et al. '*Nigella sativa* plant extract increases number and activity of immune competent cells in humans.' *Expt. Hematol.* 21, 1186 (1993).)

Dɪᴅ ʏᴏᴜ ᴋɴᴏᴡ?

❧ In Saudi Arabia, black seed is used as protection from the 'evil eye.' It is burned to produce a strong smell (external treatment) and is taken as tablets followed by water (internal treatment).

❧ Black seed was found in Tutankhamen's tomb. This suggests that black seed had an important role in ancient Egypt, since it was customary to place in tombs items needed for the afterlife.

❧ In the Old Testament, the prophet Isaiah contrasts *Nigella* (black cumin) with wheat. See Isaiah 28:25, 27.

❧ In Morocco, black seed is called *sanuj*. For coughs, asthma and other lung ailments, Moroccan herbalists recommend 3-5 drops of *sanuj* oil, taken with coffee or tea. The seed powder is taken with honey for liver or heart pain. Moroccans also use the seeds to remedy influenza, allergies, high blood pressure and stomachache.

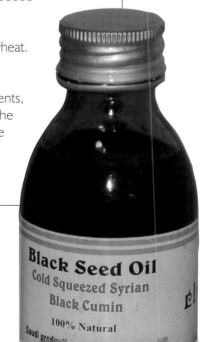

CARAWAY

Carum carvi
Apiaceae/Umbelliferae (Parsley) Family
Arabic: *karawiya*

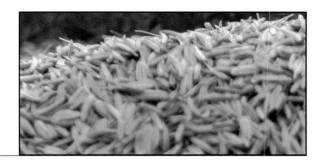

Some botanists describe caraway as the world's oldest known herb. It is mentioned in the Bible and other ancient texts, and has been found in European archaeological excavations dating back 8,000 years.

In the spice markets of Arabia, caraway can be found alongside her sister spices of anise (*yansoon*), fennel (*shamr*), and cumin (*kamun*). You need only ask for *karawiya* to take some home.

Caraway is grown throughout Europe, the Mediterranean area, North Africa, Asia and North America.

According to Dr Jabber Salem Mossa al-Kahtani, Professor and Chairman of the Department of Pharmacognosy at King Saud University, caraway is more popular in Mecca and Jeddah than in other areas of the Kingdom because pilgrims from Egypt and other parts of the Muslim world brought herbs and spices with them during the Hajj, which were adopted by Western Arabia.

HOW TO USE

1. Crush seeds to make an infusion (tea).

2. Chew whole seeds to freshen breath.

3 . Grind seeds into powder.

IN THE KITCHEN

One tablespoon of crushed caraway seeds steeped for 20 minutes in one cup of either milk or water produces a soothing drink appropriate for children and adults. Strain and sweeten with honey, if desired.

Caraway is a biennial. It grows as a small green plant the first year and then up to two feet tall the second year, producing small white and apple-green flowers and fruit. The fruit, commonly called seeds, can be separated from the plant when ripe and then dried in the sun.

RESEARCH

In a recent study, caraway was one of several herbs shown to reduce non-ulcer dyspepsia in test subjects, a development that researchers said warranted further investigation. (Thompson Coon, J., and E. Ernst. 'Systematic Review: Herbal medicinal products for non-ulcer dyspepsia.' *Alimentary Pharmacology & Therapeutics.* Volume 16 Issue 10 - October 2002.)

Another study found that essential oils in caraway seeds had potential for helping to prevent certain cancers. (Zheng, G.Q., et al. 'Anethofuran, carvone, and limonene: potential cancer chemopreventive agents from dill weed oil and caraway oil.' *Planta Med.* 1992 Aug; 58(4): 338-41.)

FAMILY REMEDIES ACROSS ARABIA

Like anise, cumin, dill and fennel, caraway is a carminative. Caraway is taken to relieve gas and to aid digestion. Both the fruit and oil possess aromatic, stimulant and carminative properties.

Breastfeeding: Caraway is used in a drink during breastfeeding to stimulate lactation. (Eastern KSA)

Colic: Caraway is used to treat colic and digestive problems in general. (KSA)

Flatulence (Intestinal Gas): Add one teaspoon of powdered caraway seeds to one cup boiling water. Steep for ten minutes and drink after meals. (KSA)

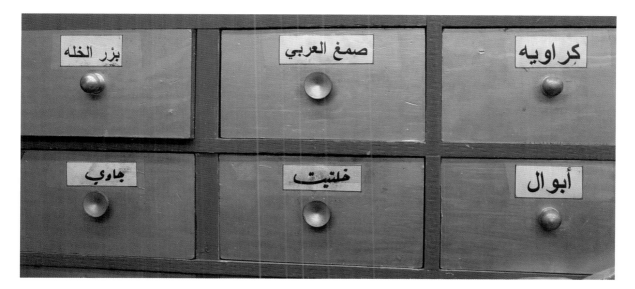

Herbal medicine chest in a Qatif shop, Saudi Arabia.

DID YOU KNOW?

᛫ Caraway seed is the spice that gives rye bread its characteristic flavour.

᛫ While best known as an important flavouring in Northern and Central European cuisines, caraway is also used in recipes of the Middle East.

᛫ Caraway is important in Tunisian cuisine, and is sometimes an ingredient of *harissa*, a fiery North African condiment made from dried hot peppers.

᛫ Caraway leaves may be used as a herb in salads and as a garnish, while its seeds may be used as a spice in breads, cheese spreads, pastas and vegetable and fruit dishes.

᛫ Dioscorides, a Greek physician in the 1st century, recommended oil of caraway be rubbed into skin to improve a pale girl's complexion.

᛫ Most experts believe the word 'caraway' comes originally from the Greek word *karon*, which means cumin! Caraway and cumin seeds are very similar in appearance. Arabic borrowed the word as *karawiya*, which medieval Latin transformed into *carui* or *carvi* (as in *Carum carvi*).

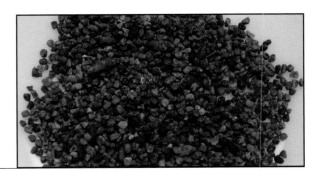

CARDAMOM

Elettaria cardamomum

Zingiberaceae (Ginger) Family

Arabic: *hal, hail*

Other English: Lesser Cardamom, Small
   Cardamom, Malabar Cardamom

Imagine an ancient trade caravan moving slowly up the Frankincense Trail in western Arabia towards the Mediterranean. The spices and aromatics burdening the camels could be from Yemen, East Africa, India or distant China. Although anticipating lucrative exchanges with merchants of the Mediterranean, caravaners also stop in villages along the way where both villagers and Bedouins are eager to barter. Exchanging goat meat, fresh produce or woven baskets, local tradesmen obtain the cardamom necessary to flavour traditional Arabic coffee.

Native to India and Sri Lanka, cardamom is a well-beloved spice in the Arabian Peninsula. Arab coffee is heavily flavoured with it. In fact, cardamom is a valuable ingredient in Middle Eastern cuisine: in beverages, sweets, pastries and main dishes.

HOW TO USE

1. Bruise cardamom pods until partially open.

2. Remove cardamom seeds from their pods. Gently bruise seeds or dry-fry over gentle heat to release their flavour.

3. Grind seeds into powder.

IN THE KITCHEN

Sweet coffee, which doesn't contain any coffee at all, is a traditional drink from the Hejaz. It is a wonderful, warm beverage with a pleasant cardamom flavour. It is served on special occasions such as graduation day for students.

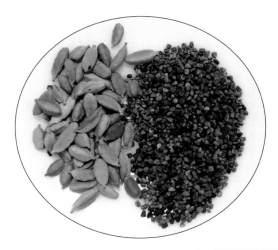

RESEARCH

Chemical analysis of some 85 commonly consumed Indian foods revealed that cardamom contains medium levels of antioxidant flavonoids (50-100 milligrams per 100 grams). (Nair, S., et al. 'Antioxidant phenolics and flavonoids in common Indian foods.' *J Assoc Physicians India.* 1998 Aug; 46(8): 708-10.)

FAMILY REMEDIES ACROSS ARABIA

A member of the ginger family, cardamom is a carminative and a stimulant. It warms the body and helps relieve indigestion and gas.

Childbirth: Following childbirth, the mother is given *jelaab*, a mixture of spices, brown flour and animal fat. *Jelaab's* spices are cardamom, ginger, black pepper, *hulwa* (fennel), cinnamon, cumin and peppermint. These spices are dried in the sun and then ground into powder. (Eastern KSA) ⬧ To strengthen the mother after childbirth, use cardamom in *aseeda*. a gruel prepared with wheat flour, dates, butter, saffron, cardamom and black pepper. (Southern KSA)

Colds and Coughs: Combine olive oil with cardamom, black seed and ginger. Heat on the fire. Rub this oil on the body. (Northern KSA)

Flatulence (Intestinal Gas): Put one teaspoon cardamom powder in a full cup of boiling water. Steep for 15 minutes and drink it three times a day after meals. (Southern KSA)

Liver: Use cardamom for the liver. (Eastern KSA)

RECIPES

Sweet Coffee, p. 180
Ghozi (Stuffed Lamb), p. 189
Hasawi Rice with Shrimp, p. 197

DID YOU KNOW?

⬧ Cardamom is one of the most expensive spices in the world. This is because each individual fruit pod containing the desired seed spice must be harvested from its flower stalk by hand. Flower stalks must be carefully examined and re-examined as the fruit pods develop at different rates. Harvested while still green and firm, the pods are then dried and sold.

⬧ About 1,000 years ago, the Vikings discovered cardamom in their explorations and conquests around the Mediterranean. They introduced this spice to Scandinavia, where it is still used extensively in baking spiced cakes and breads.

⬧ Indian cooks, in the native country of cardamom, use this spice in curries, pilafs and milky desserts.

⬧ Black cardamom *(Amomum subulatum)*, with its large brown pods, is grown in the Himalaya region, and is often described as an inferior substitute for green or true cardamom *(Elettaria cardamomum)*. In some Indian recipes they are interchangeable, but black cardamom is more often used in spicy and rustic dishes and the more subtle green cardamom in Imperial or Mughal dishes.

⬧ Cardamom was one of the most popular Oriental spices in ancient Roman cuisine – but it is believed the Romans imported black cardamom rather than green.

CASTOR OIL PLANT

Ricinus communis
Euphorbiaceae (Spurge) Family
Arabic: *khirwa', khirwa'a*

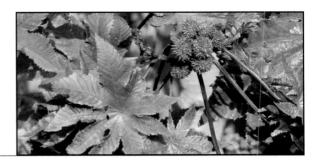

Visitors to farms in al-Hasa and areas of the Bani Hajir tribe in Saudi Arabia's Eastern Province will notice cultivation of an erect, tropical shrub or small tree whose large lobed and palmate leaves have uneven, serrated edges. Although sometimes called the castor bean plant, it is not a member of the bean family but shares the same plant family as the popular poinsettia. It is the well-known castor oil plant.

Seeds of the castor oil plant are pressed to produce castor oil, a common health store product. One of its most popular applications is the castor oil pack. This natural therapy is used for problems involving inflammation, congestion, and constipation. A castor oil pack is made of several layers of flannel wool or cotton which absorb and hold cold-pressed castor oil. Applied externally, it helps draw toxins from trouble spots within the body.

All parts of the castor plant are toxic and may produce allergic skin reactions if handled repeatedly. The seeds contain a poisonous protein called ricin. ***Just one milligram of ricin, or as few as two seeds, can kill an adult***. Symptoms of ricin poisoning in humans (abdominal pain, vomiting, diarrhoea) occur within a few hours of ingestion. If death has not resulted within 3-5 days, the victim usually recovers. Because the seeds and leaves can poison and kill, children should be kept away from this plant.

Castor oil is toxin-free when processed correctly because ricin is water-soluble and does not remain in the oil.

HOW TO USE

Apply externally to skin. Consult your physician prior to internal use.

IN THE KITCHEN

Store castor oil in a cool, dark place to prevent rancidity.

RESEARCH

Castor oil has long played a role in midwifery practice as an agent for inducing labour. In the words of Certified Professional Midwife Valerie El Halta: 'I still feel that the safest method of induction is castor oil. Many other induction methods, such as amniotomy, are irreversible and often lead to caesarean section due to "failure to progress" or time constraints for ruptured membranes. The worst things that will happen if the castor oil fails to bring on labour is the mom will have some diarrhoea and need some minerals replenished.' (*Midwifery Today*, Summer 1996, No. 38, p. 36.)

A recent clinical study of the induction effect was inconclusive, and further trials were recommended. (Kelly, A.J., et al. 'Castor oil, bath and/or enema for cervical priming and induction of labour (Cochrane Review).' *The Cochrane Library*, Issue 3, 2003.)

FAMILY REMEDIES ACROSS ARABIA

Castor oil packs do not appear to be a well-known treatment in the Kingdom. The following quotations from survey respondents reveal that castor oil has been primarily valued for cosmetic applications and stomach complaints.

Hair Loss: My mother used castor oil to prevent hair loss. (Western KSA) ❧ To prevent hair loss, use henna, garlic, castor oil, aloe and coconut. (Central KSA) ❧ For hair loss, [treat the scalp with] castor oil and henna, as well as *jarjeer* oil. (Northern KSA)

Indigestion: Boil and drink anise. Drink castor oil. (Central KSA) ❧ Use myrrh or castor oil. (Northern KSA)

Purgative: Castor bean oil is to clean the abdomen, and thyme is to clean the liver and abdomen. (Northern KSA)

Stomachache: In the past, castor bean oil, myrrh and *lisan* [possibly a variety of plantain] was used. (Northern KSA)

DID YOU KNOW?

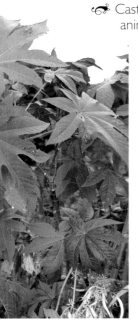

❧ Castor oil and its derivatives are used in the manufacture of soaps, lubricants, hydraulic and brake fluids, paints, dyes, inks, waxes and polishes, nylon, pharmaceuticals and perfumes.

❧ Castor meal, an organic nitrogen fertilizer, is a by-product that results when castor seeds are crushed to extract oil. With a high content of essential plant nutrients, it is an excellent organic fertilizer.

❧ Castor oil has a viscosity 20 times greater than that of any other fat or oil of vegetable or animal origin.

❧ Castor oil is an emollient known to soften and smooth tissue.

❧ Al-Kindi used leaves of the plant in a preparation to lengthen hair, in a remedy for epilepsy and in a 'preventive' clyster or enema for general good health and potency.

❧ The use of castor seed oil in India has been documented since 2000 BC for use in lamps and in local medicine as a laxative.

❧ Castor seeds have been found in Egyptian tombs dating from 4000 BC.

❧ According to Herodotus, the ancient Egyptians of the Nile delta cultivated the castor-oil plant 'along the banks of rivers and lakes' and used its oil for burning in lamps. The Greek historian said castor oil was 'quite as good as olive-oil, though the smell is unpleasant.'

❧ Castor oil is notorious for its strong taste.

CHAMOMILE

German Chamomile: Matricaria recutita,
Saudi Chamomile: Matricaria aurea,
Matricaria chamomilla
Asteraceae (Aster) Family
Arabic: *babunaj, babunij*
Other English: Camomile

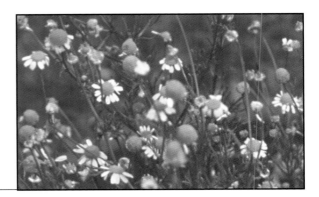

One thing every Bedouin, villager and city dweller can tell you is that chamomile tea is relaxing and aids digestion. Along with this fact comes the widespread belief that the best babunaj comes from the North. As a result, packaged herbal teas from Syria and Jordan are popular supermarket items. These medicinal teas feature chamomile but may also contain coriander, black seed, anise, rose, lemon balm, hibiscus, thyme or sage. Chamomile is also imported from Egypt. German chamomile is favoured in Saudi Arabia for its medicinal properties.

HOW TO USE

Use the flower heads to brew a medicinal tea.

IN THE KITCHEN

Many families keep chamomile readily available. To make chamomile tea, boil water and then pour one cup of the water over 4 teaspoons of dried flowers. Infuse for 5-10 minutes and then strain. Add honey for a sweeter taste and drink the tea warm.

DID YOU KNOW?

❧ In a 1937 study, anthropologist Henry Field wrote that babunaj was named after the village of Babunah in Arabia because it grew particularly abundantly there. Martin Levey, translator of al-Kindi's *Medical Formulary,* places Babunah in Persia (Iran).

❧ In 1656, John Parkinson wrote, 'Camomill is put to divers and sundry uses, both for pleasure and profit, both for the sick and the sound, in bathing to comfort and strengthen the sound and to ease pains in the diseased.'

❧ Al-Kindi used chamomile in a strong dressing for spleen and in an application to relax the liver and stomach.

❧ Chamomile tea is used in the Levant to strengthen a mother after childbirth.

❧ Applied as a plant spray, chamomile tea has been used to control a condition known as 'damping off,' a post-germination fungus disease that kills seedlings by cutting off water and nutrient intake. This disease often strikes seedlings that are planted too closely together. Spraying seedlings and soil daily with chamomile tea is a safe way to treat damping off.

FAMILY REMEDIES ACROSS ARABIA

Chamomile is a valued nervine, carminative and general tonic. Chamomile tea is well-known for settling the stomach and aiding digestion after a meal. It is also relaxing and can help promote sleep.

Colic: Soak chamomile and drink it warm without sugar. It is good for colic, relaxing, and is used as an antiseptic. (Eastern KSA) ❧ Drink chamomile tea with peppermint and anise. (Southern KSA) ❧ For babies, make a tea of cumin, peppermint, chamomile and anise. (Central KSA) ❧ From three months to one year, massage the baby's tummy with chamomile oil. (Western KSA)

Coughs: Use chamomile for coughs, chest and lung problems, as well as abdominal pains. (Eastern KSA) ❧ For coughs, drink chamomile tea with cinnamon. (Southern KSA) ❧ Take chamomile and ginger; lemon mixed with honey and black seeds; or tahina with sesame oil. Mix olive oil and ginger to rub on chest and back. (Eastern KSA)

Heart Trouble: Drink a tea of wild chamomile and cress. (Southern KSA)

Indigestion: Make an infusion from a dried herb mixture of chamomile, green tea, peppermint and basil. (Southern KSA)

Menstrual Pain: Chamomile, the medicinal kind that grows in Syria and in the Levant, is used to treat stomachaches, menstrual pain and coughs. Place one-half spoonful of chamomile flowers in a *finjan* and add hot water. Let sit for five minutes. Don't drink more than two *finjan* every day. (Eastern KSA) ❧ Drink chamomile tea. (Central KSA) ❧ Chamomile, cinnamon, cloves [in a tea]. (Northern KSA)

Stomachache: Infuse a mixture of chamomile, cane sugar and mint with water and drink. (UAE)

Stress: Chamomile and anise tea helps you relax. (Central KSA) ❧ Chamomile is for relaxing the nerves, inducing sleep and cleansing the body internally. (Northern KSA)

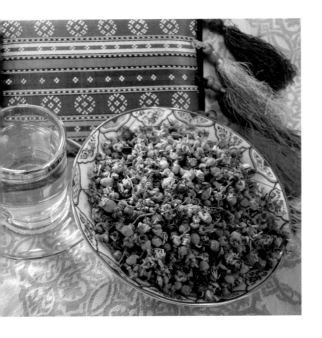

RESEARCH

A compound of apple pectin and chamomile has been shown to be effective in controlling diarrhoea in children. (De la Mott, S., et al. '[Double-blind comparison of an apple pectin-chamomile extract preparation with placebo in children with diarrhoea].' *Arzneimittelforschung.* 1997 Nov;47(11):1247-9.)

A chamomile-based ointment Kamillosan has been shown to be superior to hydrocortisone for treatment of contact dermatitis. (Nissen, H.P., et al. '[Profilometry, a method for the assessment of the therapeutic effectiveness of Kamillosan ointment].' *Z Hautkr.* 1988 Mar 21;63(3):184-90.)

CINNAMON

Cinnamomum zeylanicum or C.ceylanicum or C.verum
Lauraceae Family
Arabic: *qurfa, qirfah, darsini*
Other English: Ceylon Cinnamon

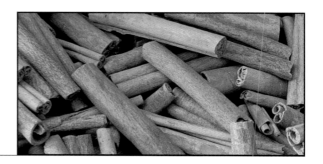

For at least 5,000 years Arabian peoples dominated the movement of spices. A glance at a map of ancient trade routes reveals why. The Arabs were geographically poised to receive spices from the East and then transport and sell them to merchants in North Africa and around the Mediterranean. To maintain their trade monopoly and keep prices high, Arab tradesmen obscured the origin of the spices by telling tall tales. Herodotus (5th century BC) relates:

> The Arabians say that the dry sticks, which we call kinamomon, are brought to Arabia by large birds, which carry them to their nests, made of mud, on mountain precipices which no man can climb. The method invented to get the cinnamon sticks is this. People cut up the bodies of dead oxen into very large joints, and leave them on the ground near the nests. They then scatter, and the birds fly down and carry off the meat to their nests, which are too weak to bear the weight and fall to the ground. The men come and pick up the cinnamon. Acquired in this way, it is exported to other countries.

Not everyone believed the tales. Pliny the Elder (AD 23-79) wrote in *Natural History*: 'Those old tales were invented by the Arabians to raise the price of their goods.' Nevertheless, the exact source of cinnamon remained a mystery through the Middle Ages. In the late 14th century, the renowned traveller Ibn Battuta revealed the island of Sri Lanka to be a source of cinnamon. He explained that people from southern India came to Sri Lanka to collect cinnamon and then later dealt with traders from elsewhere.

Emerging European sea powers raced to find sea routes to the East. The Portuguese took control of the Spice Islands in the early 1500s, were ousted by the Dutch in 1605, and later the British assumed control. The Arabs' spice trade monopoly was gone forever.

HOW TO USE

Use cinnamon sticks whole or grind into powder.

IN THE KITCHEN

In Middle Eastern cuisine, powdered cinnamon flavours desserts such as *Muhallabiyya*, a milk pudding, and *Umm 'Ali*, a dish made from old flat bread and milk with sugar and cinnamon. Although originally introduced from Egypt, *Umm 'Ali* is very popular in Saudi Arabia. In traditional Arab dishes, such as ground-meat favourites kofta and kibbeh, cinnamon is known to improve meat flavour. Cinnamon sticks are added whole to rice dishes and soup.

Cinnamon should be stored in an airtight jar and kept in a cool, dark cupboard.

RECIPES

Date Bars, p. 200
Hasawi Rice with Shrimp, p. 197
Mufallaq with Meat, p. 196
Wheat Soup, p. 187

RESEARCH

Cinnamon shows promise in fighting Candida (yeast) oral infections in HIV patients. (Quale, J.M. et al. 'In vitro activity of Cinnamomum zeylanicum against azole resistant and sensitive Candida species and a pilot study of cinnamon for oral candidiasis.' *Am J Chin Med*. 1996; 24 (2): 103-9.)

Recent research in India shows that cinnamon exerts significant antioxidant protection of the heart and liver in rats on a high-fat diet. (Dhuley, J.N. 'Anti-oxidant effects of cinnamon (Cinnamomum verum) bark and greater cardamom (Amomum subulatum) seeds in rats fed high fat diet.' *Indian J Exp Biol*. 1999 Mar; 37(3): 238-42.)

FAMILY REMEDIES ACROSS ARABIA

A marvelous variety of cinnamon tea applications surfaced in the 2002 survey. Unique combinations of ingredients are reported.

Childbirth: Boil 2-3 cinnamon sticks and drink liquid (remove sticks) for relief of menstrual pain or when you feel contractions before delivery. (Western KSA) ⋙ Boil cinnamon or cloves with honey and eat dates during labour. (Central KSA) ⋙ To make the delivery faster and easier, drink boiled cinnamon. (Central & Northern KSA) ⋙ In the past they used *jelaab* – ginger, black pepper, fennel, cinnamon, cumin, cardamom and peppermint – dried in the sun and ground. (Central KSA) ⋙ Use dates, *bukhoor* of *'ud*, cinnamon and cumin. (Central KSA) ⋙ After delivery, drink cinnamon tea, coffee bean peelings tea, and boiled sheep's milk. (Southern KSA) ⋙ Make an infusion of cinnamon and a natural mixture of flowers (roses). (Southern KSA) ⋙ Drink cinnamon and eat *aseeda* (flour blended with fat and dates) to strengthen the mother. (Southern KSA) ⋙ To strengthen the mother after childbirth, use fenugreek, cress, black seeds, cumin, cinnamon, whole-wheat flour with honey and butter, and *thareed*, a dish with vegetables, tomato sauce, and meat with small pieces of bread. (Central KSA) ⋙ After delivery, take fenugreek, cress, cinnamon, sage and peppermint. (Central KSA)

Colds or Coughs: Use cinnamon and chamomile. (Southern KSA) ⋙ For colds, use ginger and cinnamon. (Southern KSA)

Menstrual Pain: Mix sage with cinnamon and boil, or use cinnamon, dried limes, and olive oil. (Western KSA) ⋙ Boil cinnamon and ginger for 25 minutes and drink. (Western KSA) ⋙ Drink hot peppermint and cinnamon – and a tea made from coffee bean peelings. Cinnamon helps to stimulate the menses if a period is late. (Southern KSA) ⋙ Boil cinnamon, ginger and mint and drink (Northern KSA) ⋙ Use chamomile, cinnamon, cumin and cloves. Cinnamon is for inflammation of the uterus. (Northern KSA) ⋙ For cramps, drink cinnamon boiled in water. (Eastern KSA & UAE) ⋙ Use mint, cinnamon, chamomile, *loomi* and sage boiled with water. (Central KSA)

Stomachache: Drink cinnamon tea. (KSA) ⋙ For stomachaches, boil and sweeten cinnamon and sage. (Bahrain) ⋙ Use cinnamon, cumin and anise. (Southern KSA) ⋙ Drink mint and cinnamon (boiled in water) as hot drinks. (Eastern KSA) ⋙ Use dates, honey and boiled cinnamon. (Eastern KSA)

DID YOU KNOW?

⋙ Cinnamon has one of the oldest known histories. Moses used it as an ingredient in holy anointing oils (Exodus 30:22-25).

⋙ Egyptian Queen Cleopatra (69-30 BC) carried cinnamon with her jewels.

⋙ Celebrated physician and translator Hunayn ibn Ishaq (died 873) lists cinnamon as an eye remedy.

⋙ *Cinnamomum zeylanicum* is regarded by some as a folk-remedy abortifacient for unwanted pregnancies.

⋙ Cinnamon is an aromatic, carminative, astringent and stimulant. It is said to counter edema and jaundice. It is considered an antidote for upset stomachs worldwide.

CLOVE

Syzygium aromaticum (also *Caryophyllus
    aromaticus* and *Eugenia aromatica*)
Myrtaceae (Myrtle) Family
Arabic: *qaranful, mismar*

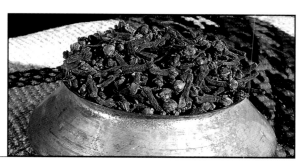

W ars have been fought over this spice, the unopened flower buds of a tropical evergreen tree. Consider Manuel, King of Portugal, in the early 1500s. Consumers in his country and throughout Europe were demanding greater quantities of spices. Manuel's merchant ships travelled to Mediterranean ports to trade with Arabs who brought spices from the East. Arabian peoples had monopolized the spice trade for centuries, and King Manuel was determined to gain control of the trade. He sent fleets around Africa to India and East Africa in a move to strengthen Portuguese influence. In 1511, he sent an expedition to conquer Meleka, a commercial centre in what is now Malaysia. His fleet was victorious and continued eastwards to claim the Spice Islands, home of the famed clove tree.

Through their supremacy at sea, the Portuguese ended Arab domination of the spice trade and ruled over the Spice Islands throughout the 16th century. So valuable was the clove trade that in 1605 the Dutch waged a successful war with the Portuguese for control of it.

In the mid-1700s, a Frenchman, Pierre Poivre (Peter Pepper), stole some clove trees from the Dutch-controlled Spice Islands and

began to produce cloves in present-day Mauritius. From there, clove trees were shipped to other French territories such as Bourbon Island (now Reunion) in the Indian Ocean and Martinique in the Caribbean.

Today, clove-producing areas include the islands east of Africa (Mauritius, Zanzibar, Pemba, and Madagascar), Brazil, and the islands of Indonesia, the original Spice Islands.

HOW TO USE

1. Use cloves whole.

2. Grind into powder.

IN THE KITCHEN

Cloves are abundantly available in traditional herb and spice markets as well as in modern supermarkets throughout the Middle East. Says a resident of the Eastern Province (KSA): 'We use cumin, coriander, black pepper, cinnamon, parsley, mint and cloves as spices and herbs for cooking.'

| RECIPES | *Mufallaq with Meat, p. 196* |

DID YOU KNOW?

❧ In the 3rd century BC visitors to the emperor of China were required to chew a clove in advance of the meeting in order not to have offensive breath.

❧ Al-Kindi used clove in a dentifrice for treating rotten teeth and bad breath, in a collyrium (eye wash or eye salve) that improves vision, and in a drug that strengthens breathing.

❧ Clove cigarettes, or *kreteks*, consisting of two parts tobacco to one part cloves, are popular in Indonesia and consume much of the world's crop.

FAMILY REMEDIES ACROSS ARABIA

Throughout history, physicians have found cloves very useful for a wide range of ailments. The aromatic clove is a carminative and stimulant. It warms the body, increases circulation, improves digestion, and treats flatulence, vomiting and nausea. It is also an antiseptic and mildly anesthetic. Its properties validate its use in many of the following remedies:

Coughs or Colds: Take cloves in honey. (Northern KSA) ❧ Heat olive oil and cloves and rub it on the body. (Northern KSA)

Cuts: Cloves were used on wounds in the past. Now, people use different disinfectants. (Central KSA)

Childbirth: Use boiled cinnamon or cloves with honey and eat dates during labour. (Central KSA)

Eyes: For a small abscess in the rim or inner corner of the eye, chew a clove to soften it, then poke it into the abscess until it bleeds. Chew another clove and rub it into the bleeding area. (Socotra, Yemen) ❧ For an opaque cornea, grind a clove and put the powder in the eye to 'suck out the disease'. (Socotra, Yemen)

Hair Loss: Mix cloves, salt and henna. Use every two weeks or monthly. (Northern KSA)

Headaches: Use ground cloves with olive oil and put it on the afflicted area of the head while warm. (Central KSA) ❧ In the past, olive oil, cloves, henna, and fenugreek were heated on the stove and put on the head. (Northern KSA) ❧ Mix powdered black seed with one-half of the amount of powdered cloves and one-half of the amount of anise. Eat this mixture with a spoonful of yoghurt. Also, apply black seed oil on the painful area. (Eastern KSA)

Menstrual Cramps: Use boiled cumin and boiled cloves with honey. (Central KSA) ❧ Take chamomile, cinnamon and cloves. (Northern KSA)

Nausea and Vomiting: Boil cloves with black seeds and drink without sweeteners three times a day. This is good for vomiting and nausea. You may not need the third dose. (Eastern KSA)

Sore Throat: Boil cloves and ginger in water and drink it to help soothe a sore throat. (UAE)

Toothache: Apply ground cloves on aching teeth to reduce pain. (Eastern KSA) ❧ Use cloves for tooth pain. (Central KSA)

RESEARCH

Antibacterial and fungicidal activity has been noted in clove oil. The fungus control properties were significant enough to warrant recommending clove oil as a safe and natural post-harvest treatment for bananas affected by fungal damage. (Ranasinghe, L. 'Fungicidal activity of essential oils of *Cinnamomum zeylanicum* and *Syzygium aromaticum*'; Merr (L.) et L. M. Perry. 'Against crown rot and anthracnose pathogens isolated from banana.' *Lett Appl Microbiol.* 2002; 35(3):208-11; Burt, S.A., and R.D. Reinders. 'Antibacterial activity of selected plant essential oils against Escherichia coli O157:H7.' *Lett Appl Microbiol.* 2003; 36(3):162-7.)

COFFEE

Coffea arabica, C. robusta, et al.
Rubiaceae (Madder) Family
Arabic: *qahwa, bunn*

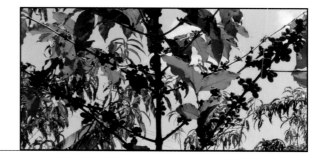

The lore surrounding the coffee bean and the amazing beverage derived from it goes back thousands of years. According to one legend, a young man named Kaldi lived in Abyssinia (Ethiopia) around 300 BC. While tending his goats, he noticed them frolicking more than usual. At first perplexed, he soon realized their friskiness was caused by eating the bright red berries from a nearby shrub. Hearing this, monks at a local monastery created a drink from the berries and found they could stay more alert during prayers. Experimentation with burning and grinding the berries led to the discovery of the black beverage we know today as coffee.

By the 15th century, the coffee plant, which grew wild in Ethiopia, was being cultivated in Yemen. Over the next two centuries, Yemen supplied the world with coffee. The Yemenis had a policy of not exporting fertile beans, so that coffee could not be cultivated anywhere else. But the resourceful Dutch somehow obtained coffee seedlings from Mocha, Yemen, in the early 17th century and introduced the plant to Ceylon (Sri Lanka), India and Dutch Asian colonies such as Java and Sumatra. Yemen lost its monopoly on coffee production and trade, and the Dutch became the main suppliers to Europe.

In Arabia, hospitality is incomplete without *qahwah*. Serving freshly brewed coffee has for centuries been a way to welcome and honour guests. Traditionally, green coffee beans are lightly roasted over a fire in a long-handled utensil called a *mihmas*. They are stirred often, so they do not turn too dark and bitter. The roasted beans are placed in a wooden coffee box to cool and later ground with a mortar and pestle, ready to boil into a cup of coffee.

HOW TO USE

1. Remove husks before roasting coffee beans.

2. Use coffee beans whole or grind into powder.

IN THE KITCHEN

Cardamom is a vital ingredient in Arabian coffee. Its flavour is added to the beverage by grinding cardamom pods and adding the powder to already brewed coffee. Cloves, saffron, sugar, *nakhwa* (*ajwain*) or rose water are also sometimes added for flavour.

HOW TO SERVE

A host holds the coffee pot in his left hand and the small coffee cups stacked in his right hand while walking around to serve guests. He serves guests of honour or those highest in rank first. Otherwise, he serves guests according to seating, proceeding from right to left. It is considered bad manners to give or receive anything using the left hand, so a guest should be careful to accept coffee cups only with the right hand.

Coffee traditions are passed from one generation to the next. Generally, a server should fill a cup one-third full or just less than half. This way, the coffee does not get cold. The server should watch closely and immediately refill cups as needed. It is bad manners for a guest to put a coffee cup on a table or on the floor. When the guest has had enough coffee, the proper step is to shake the empty cup with small back and forth movements of the wrist. The server will then remove the cup.

Notes a Saudi respondent: 'Coffee has a special, delicious taste and you can think more clearly and sometimes find solutions to problems when you drink coffee. When you visit most people, they feel it's necessary to prepare and serve a cup of coffee or tea. It is the basis of all parties.'

FAMILY REMEDIES ACROSS ARABIA

The best-known medicinal use of coffee, in Arabia and the rest of the world, is as a brain stimulant that produces alertness and sometimes sleeplessness. But Arabian traditional medicine has found many other uses as well.

Abdominal Pain: Coffee beans are cooked and the resulting coffee water is used as a drink to lessen abdominal pain. (Southern KSA)

Appetite: To restore a lost appetite, drink strong coffee and then wash in hot water. (Socotra, Yemen).

Bleeding: Ground coffee is to be put on fresh open wounds as temporary first aid until you get to the hospital. (Western KSA) ❧ Coffee and salt on wounds is to stop bleeding. (Northern KSA) ❧ Ground coffee is put on a bleeding wound to help the blood to clot and stop the bleeding. (Southern KSA)

Childbirth: To strengthen a mother after childbirth, drink cinnamon, coffee bean husks, and boiled sheep milk. (Southern KSA)

Diarrhoea: Use a mixture of coffee and grated onion and one spoon of honey. Take one *finjan* to stop diarrhoea. (Eastern KSA)

Eyes: Coffee is for sore eyes. (Northern KSA)

Headaches: Drink coffee. (Central KSA)

Menstrual Pain: For cramps, drink hot peppermint and cinnamon – and coffee bean husks. (Southern KSA)

Nausea: Drink strong coffee to relieve nausea, settle the stomach and restore the appetite. (Socotra, Yemen)

Sore Throats: Myrrh and coffee. Gargle with hot water and salt. (Southern KSA)

Stomachaches: Drink Arabic coffee. (Southern KSA)

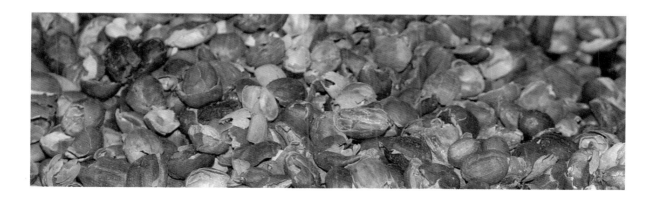

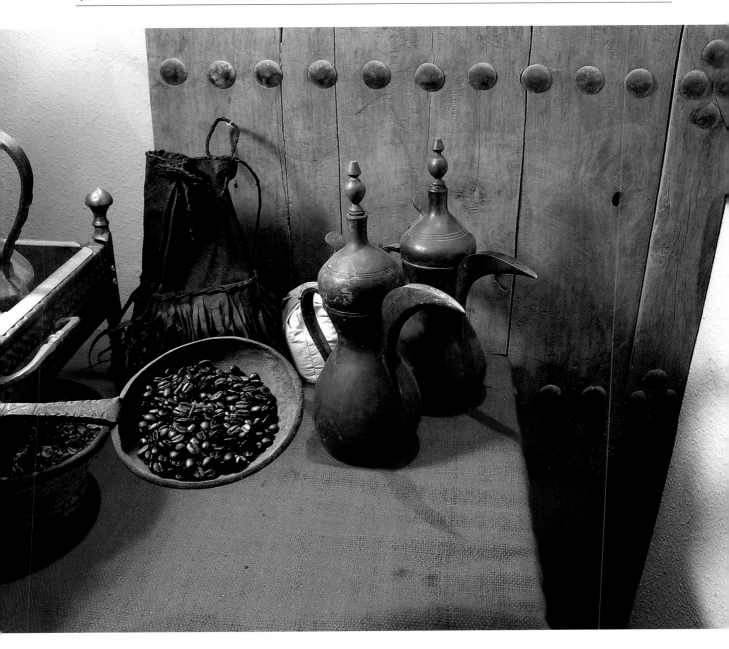

RESEARCH

Brewed coffee contains many antioxidants and may inhibit diseases caused by oxidative damage, according to a study by the University of California at Davis and the Japan Institute for Control of Aging. (Yanagimoto, K., et al. 'Antioxidative activities of fractions obtained from brewed coffee.' *J Agric Food Chem*. 2004 Feb 11 ;52(3): 592-6.)

Drinking coffee may favourably affect cardiovascular health by decreasing LDL cholesterol and reducing LDL oxidation susceptibility, scientists in Japan report. (Yukawa, G.S., et al. 'Effects of coffee consumption on oxidative susceptibility of low-density lipoproteins and serum lipid levels in humans.' *Biochemistry (Mosc)*. 2004 Jan; 69(1): 70-4.)

DID YOU KNOW?

🐛 There are some 40 species of the *Coffea* genus, the two most popular being *arabica* and *robusta*. The *arabica* bean is harder than *robusta*, and is generally considered superior because of its full body and rich flavour.

🐛 The coffee plant produces small, red, berry-like fruits, each containing two seeds or beans, wrapped in husks or 'parchment'. In Arabic, the fruit itself is called *bunn*, while the coffee bean and its husk, are called *bunn (or habb al-bunn)* and *qishr* respectively.

🐛 The coffee industry provides employment for millions of people worldwide. It is crucial to the economies of many developing countries, such as Cameroon, Tanzania, Uganda and Ivory Coast.

🐛 In the Ayurvedic tradition, unripe coffee beans have been used to treat headaches while the ripe, roasted beans have been used for diarrhoea.

🐛 The Turks of the Ottoman Empire, who controlled parts of Eastern Europe in their day, are believed to have introduced Europeans to coffee. The famed dark roasts of present-day Vienna are said to be a result of that city's closeness to Ottoman frontiers in the 16th century.

🐛 Coffee houses were popular meeting places in colonial New York, Philadelphia and Boston. The Boston Tea Party of 1773 was planned in a coffee house, the Green Dragon.

RECIPES

Arabic Coffee, p. 178
Arabic Coffee with Nakhwa, p. 179
Omani Coffee, p. 181

Grinding coffee, in a Bedouin tent display, Eastern Province, Saudi Arabia.

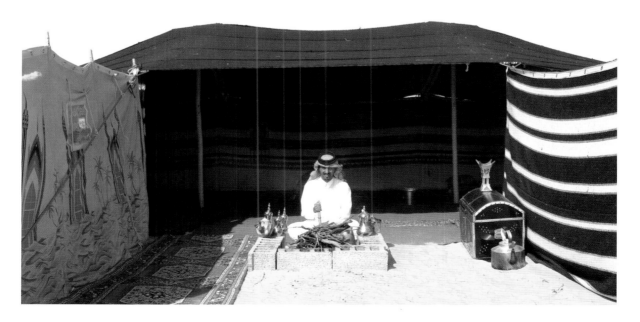

CORIANDER

Coriandrum sativum L.
Apiaceae/Umbelliferae (Parsley) Family
Arabic: *kuzbara, kizbara*
Other English: (leaves) Cilantro, Chinese
  Parsley

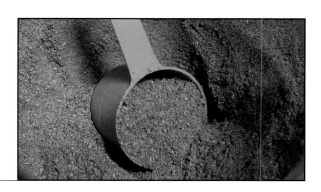

This versatile plant produces both an herb and a spice. The leaves are the herb and are known as cilantro or Chinese parsley; its round seeds are the spice coriander. The Arabic word for coriander, *kuzbara*, refers to both its seeds and its leaves.

In present-day Iran, coriander seeds are smoked like tobacco to relieve toothaches, and an infusion of the leaves is said to remedy headaches.

Coriander is a major herbal crop in Morocco, Romania and Egypt, and is also grown in China and India.

HOW TO USE

1. Use seeds in whole spice mixtures.

2. Grind seeds to use in powdered spice mixtures.

3. Use fresh leaves in salads, soups and meat dishes.

IN THE KITCHEN

Fresh coriander leaves (cilantro) flavour dishes such as salad, lentil soup and lamb. Coriander seeds are an important ingredient in *baharat*, an Arabic spice mixture often used to flavour meat *kabsa* as well as other dishes. Dry-frying the seeds prior to use greatly enhances flavour.

| RECIPE | *Mufallaq with Meat, p. 196* |

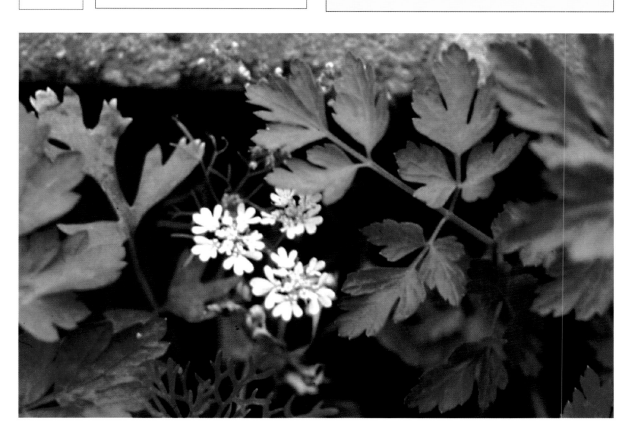

FAMILY REMEDIES ACROSS ARABIA

Coriander is considered healthful for the body. It is also an ingredient in mixed herb teas sold in the markets. As a carminative, it serves to aid digestion. Coriander seeds can be roasted and boiled with fresh ginger, then strained, and the liquid used to relieve flu symptoms.

Digestion: Pour water that has been brought to a boil over a teaspoon of coriander seed powder. Steep for ten minutes. Drink this liquid three times a day following meals. (Southern KSA)

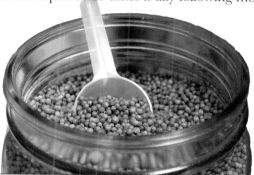

DID YOU KNOW?

☙ In the Old Testament, manna is likened to a coriander seed (Exodus16:31; Numbers 11:7).

☙ Coriander was grown in ancient Persia, and was also cultivated for its fragrance in the hanging gardens of Babylon.

☙ Coriander seeds were found in the tombs of the Pharaohs. The ancient Egyptians used the seeds to treat head pain and other head ailments. Today's Egyptians use coriander as a carminative, stomachic, digestive and culinary condiment.

☙ Hippocrates (400 BC) recommended coriander as a general tonic.

☙ Indian cooking calls for large quantities of coriander in curry powders, *garam masala*, and other spice mixes.

☙ Spanish conquistadors introduced coriander/cilantro to Mexico and Peru, where it now commonly accompanies chilies in the local cuisine.

☙ In Yemeni cookery, a thick spicy paste called *zhoug* (or *zhug*) contains both coriander leaves and fruits, in addition to green chili, garlic, cardamom and black pepper. It may also include cumin, lemon juice and olive oil. *Zhoug* is served as a relish or bread dip.

RESEARCH

Scientists have studied the antimicrobial activity of coriander seed oil and cilantro leaf oil. Cilantro oil has been shown to be particularly effective against Listeria bacteria. (Delaquis, P.J., et al. 'Antimicrobial activity of individual and mixed fractions of dill, cilantro, coriander and eucalyptus essential oils.' *Int J Food Microbiol.* 2002 Mar 25; 74(1-2): 101-9.)

CRESS

Lepidium sativum
Brassicaceae (Cabbage) Family
Arabic: *rashad, rishad, hilf, al-hara*
Other English: Garden Cress, Pepperweed,
Peppergrass

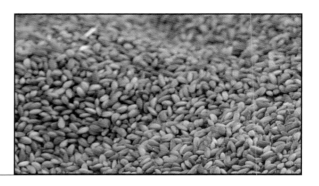

P icture this scene over 150 years ago: a small group on camelback is crossing the desolate sands near Tabuk in northwest Arabia. Finnish explorer Georg Wallin and his guides are making their way south. Suddenly, the travellers encounter a plain of green, as far as the eye can see:

> We entered a plain of soft sand, called al-Mahîr, which was exuberant of pasture as the other was barren. It lay before us one sheet of verdure, being covered with a plant called *al-hârrâ*, of a bitter but very pleasant taste, something like our cresses. This is a pasture of which the camel is very fond. When dried it is also used as a stomachic by the Arabs of the towns, who then called it *rishâd*.

Cress is cultivated in the peninsula today (in Taif, Abha and Qasim, for example) since its seed (sometimes known as red seed) is valued as medicine. It is occasionally found growing as a weed in the coastal lowlands of Saudi Arabia's Eastern Province. Indeed, the plant grows wild from Sudan to the Himalayas. It is thought to be native to Western Asia (perhaps Iran), but spread many centuries ago to Europe and the rest of Asia.

Cress is an annual, erect herbaceous plant, which grows up to 50 centimetres. It is well-suited to all types of soils and climates, although it does not tolerate frosts.

HOW TO USE

1. Grind the seeds to powder and use in food.

2. Eat the seeds whole.

3. Boil the seeds in water and drink.

IN THE KITCHEN

Cress leaves can add a delicious peppery taste to salads. Cress owes its delicate aroma to health-promoting isothiocyanates. Since isothiocyanates are volatile and susceptible to heat and moisture, cress leaves should not be dried or cooked.

Cress seeds (*rashad*) are mixed with brown flour and animal fat to strengthen a mother after childbirth. A dish called al-Hesou, or spicy flour pudding with eggs, features *rashad* for this purpose.

RECIPE

*Spicy Flour Pudding
with Eggs (Al-Hesou), p. 202*

FAMILY REMEDIES ACROSS ARABIA

Cress seeds (*rashad*) are sold in local herb shops and are used for medicinal purposes. As one resident of Central Saudi Arabia puts it: '*Rashad* is used for muscle relaxation and it helps when you are shedding hair. It also helps asthma and apnea and stimulates menstruation and cleans and cures the lungs.'

Blood Cleanser: Mix 1 spoon of *rashad* with 1 egg, 1 glass of milk, and 1 spoon of honey to cleanse the blood. (Western KSA)

Boils: *Rashad* is used for boils. (Southern KSA)

Broken Bones: Eat the seeds, powdered or whole, or the leaves to speed up the healing of broken bones. (Eastern KSA)

Coughs: Drink frankincense soaked with a little myrrh and also use *rashad* for coughs. (Central KSA)

Childbirth: Use red seed to strengthen a mother after childbirth. (UAE) ᔬ Grind *rashad* and use in food as a treatment for women after delivery. (Central KSA) ᔬ Fenugreek and *rashad* (cress seed) and black pepper are good after delivery. (Central KSA) ᔬ Use black seed with honey, *rashad*, and fenugreek. Together they are used as a medication for stomachache and after giving birth, taken twice a day. (Eastern KSA) ᔬ Red seed (*rashad* or cress) is similar to black seed and is used in a soup

Fenugreek (left) and cress (right) in a herb shop in Qatif, Saudi Arabia. *Continued overleaf*

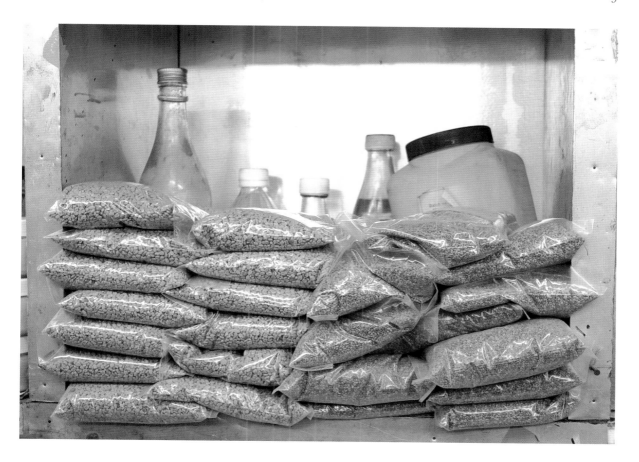

FAMILY REMEDIES ACROSS ARABIA

to strengthen the back and womb. (Southern KSA) ⅋ Use fenugreek, *rashad*, black seeds, cumin, cinnamon, whole-wheat flour with honey and butter, meat and *thareed*, a dish with vegetables, tomato sauce, and meat with small pieces of bread. (Central KSA) ⅋ Cook *rashad* seeds in hot water and sugar and drink to strengthen the back. (Southern KSA) ⅋ Use fenugreek, *rashad* and black seeds as well as cumin, black pepper and ginger. (Northern KSA) ⅋ Eat cooked wheat, protein from meat, chicken and eggs, vegetable soup, and honey and black seed with boiled eggs. Also use fenugreek and *rashad*. (Eastern KSA) ⅋ Take fenugreek, cress, cinnamon, sage and peppermint. (Eastern KSA) ⅋ Use fenugreek, *rashad*, myrrh and *laban*. (Eastern KSA)

Diabetes: Mix 1 tablespoon of myrrh, 1 cup of *rashad*, $1/2$ cup of black seed, $1/2$ cup of ground pomegranate, 1 cup of ground dried cabbage root, and a small spoon of cumin seeds. Eat this on an empty stomach, or with yogurt to make it easier to eat. It is good for diabetes. (Eastern KSA)

Hair Loss: Use *rashad* and henna. (Central KSA)

Indigestion: Use honey, *jarjeer* (arugula), *karrath* (leeks), dates and *rashad*. Mix the dates with *rashad* and a little butter and eat it while warm – it's very nourishing. (Central KSA)

Kidney Stones: Use the small red seeds of *hilf* (*rashad*) to treat kidney stones. (Yemen)

Sore Throats: Take ginger, *rashad* and myrrh. (Central KSA)

Stomachache: Take black seed with honey, *rashad* and fenugreek twice a day. (Eastern KSA) ⅋ Use fenugreek, *rashad*, cinnamon, peppermint and sage. (Eastern KSA)

DID YOU KNOW?

⌁ Xenophon, a pupil of Socrates (400 BC), mentions that the Persians used to eat cress even before bread was known.

⌁ The ancient Spartans ate cress leaves with bread. Cress is still enjoyed today with bread and butter.

⌁ During the Middle Ages, cress enjoyed prestige on royal tables. The young leaves were used for salads.

⌁ Andalusian agronomists of the Middle Ages (Ibn Hayyay, Ibn Wafid, Ibn al-Baytar, Ibn Luyun, Ibn al-Awwam) and doctors, such as Maimonides, mention garden cress. Cress was recognized as an antiscorbutic, depurative and stimulant.

⌁ Ibn Massa stated that cress relieves colic and gets rid of tapeworms and other intestinal worms.

⌁ Ibn al-Baytar reported that if hair is washed with garden cress water, it is 'purified' and hair loss is minimized.

⌁ Cress was used as an insect repellent during the Middle Ages.

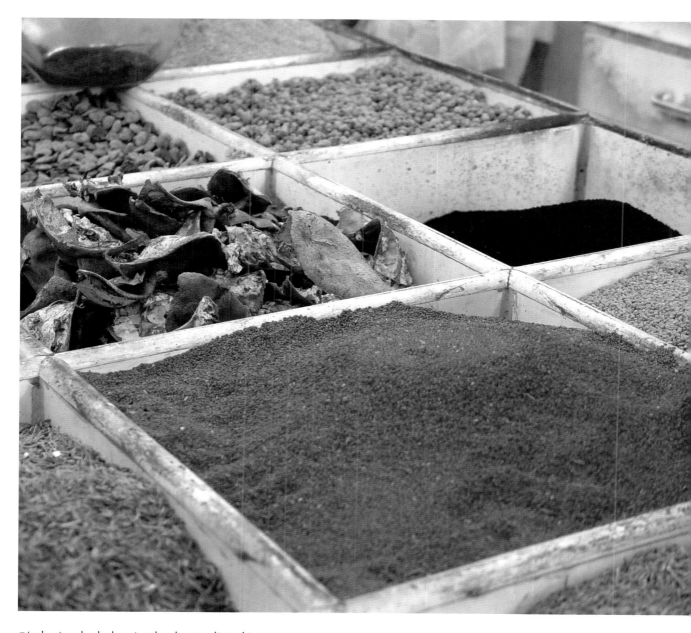

Display in a herb shop in Thuqba, Saudi Arabia.

RESEARCH

Rashad contains chemicals called isothiocyanates, found in many members of the Cabbage family, which help to fight lung and oesophageal cancer. Studies suggest that risks of cancer of the gastrointestinal and respiratory tracts can also be reduced by consuming isothiocyanate-rich vegetables. (London S.J., et al. 'Isothiocyanates, glutathione S-transferase M1 and T1 polymorphisms, and lung cancer risk: a prospective study of men in Shanghai, China.' *Lancet* 2000; 356 (9231): 724-9. Hecht, S.S. 'Inhibition of carcinogenesis by isothiocyanates.' *Drug Metab Rev* 2000; 32:395-411. Edens, N.K. 'Representative components of functional food science.' *Nutr Today*; July 1999.)

CUCUMBER

Cucumis sativus
Cucurbitaceae (Gourd) Family
Arabic: *khiyar*

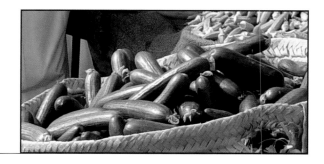

Cucumbers are produced on small farms throughout the Arabian Peninsula and sold in local fruit and vegetable markets. They have long been known in Eastern and Western traditional medicine as one of the best natural diuretics. The effect is in the seeds, which are rich in sulphur, silicon and potassium.

Cucumbers originated in Asia, probably in India, and spread into Europe about 3,000 years ago. Today Indian medicine prescribes cucumber juice for an array of ailments, including constipation, stomach disorders, urinary problems, rheumatism and even cholera.

RECIPES

Fattoush, p. 185
Tabbouleh, p. 184
Cucumber Yoghurt Salad, p. 183
Cucumber and Tomato Salad, p. 183

HOW TO USE

1. Slice or finely chop the cucumber to add to salads.

2. Slice, grate or mash the cucumber for use in skin care applications.

IN THE KITCHEN

Middle Eastern cuisine would not be the same without the cucumber. Traditional salads, such as *fattoush* and *tabbouleh*, call for this fruit posing as a vegetable, as does the popular yogurt and cucumber salad, which complements and cools rice and meat dishes. Sliced cucumbers and tomatoes, drizzled with lemon juice and garnished with fresh mint and parsley, form the renowned cucumber and tomato salad. Arranged decoratively on a serving plate, it is a simple yet healthy choice.

Did you know?

❧ The cucumber is native to India. It was a popular food in ancient Rome, and historian Pliny the Elder reports that the Emperor Tiberius ate large quantities of cucumbers.

❧ The cucumber is a fruit because it contains the seeds to reproduce. Botanically speaking, a fruit is the mature ovary of a plant, such as a cucumber, apple, melon or tomato.

❧ Cucumbers, along with squash, melons and pumpkins, belong to the group of vegetables known as cucurbits, or vine crops.

❧ Nicholas Culpeper, the 17th-century English physician who wrote *The Complete Herbal*, recommends cucumber juice for cleansing the skin, treating sunburn and fading freckles. He also cites use of the juice and seeds for promoting urine flow and healing ulcers of the bladder.

FAMILY REMEDIES ACROSS ARABIA

Suparna Trikha, one of India's leading natural beauty experts, offered advice to women of the Arabian Peninsula in the April 20-26, 2001, edition of *Friday* magazine, produced by *Gulf News* in Dubai (UAE). She stated that the juice made from cucumber skin can be a soothing lotion and skin cleanser. She also suggested grating cucumber and massaging the pulp into the skin and leaving it to dry. Splashing fresh water and gently wiping the face after ten minutes or so is a good way to slow the advance of wrinkles.

The following are reported uses of cucumber throughout the peninsula:

Eyes: Cucumber slices are put on swollen eyes, to reduce the swelling. (Eastern KSA)

Indigestion: Eating cucumber can relieve heartburn. (Eastern KSA)

Insomnia: If you have trouble sleeping, use yoghurt, cucumber or apple. (Central KSA)

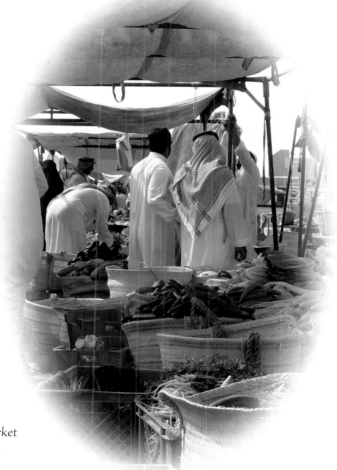

Outdoor vegetable market at al-Hasa, Saudi Arabia.

RESEARCH

Cucumber was one of 12 edible plants tested on rabbits that showed a significant ability to reduce blood sugar levels, suggesting a possible role in preventing diabetes mellitus. (Roman-Ramos, R., et al. 'Anti-hyperglycemic effect of some edible plants.' *J Ethnopharmacol* 1995 Aug 11; 48(1): 25-32.)

CUMIN

Cuminum cyminum
Apiaceae/Umbelliferae (Parsley) Family
Arabic: *kammun*
Other English: Green Cumin, White
Cumin, Cummin, Comino

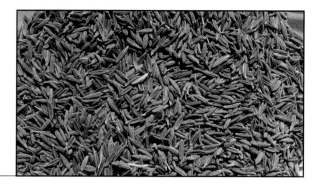

History comes alive as we trace the movement of cumin. Native to the Nile Valley, it naturally spread to neighbouring countries of northern Africa, the Mediterranean, and east to Asia where warm weather and direct sunlight provide ideal growing conditions. In the 8th century AD, the Moors (Muslims of northwest Africa) conquered southern Spain, introducing cumin there too.

Spanish explorers later carried cumin to Mexico in the New World, where it remains tremendously popular in many dishes, including tamales, tacos, salsas, sauces and soups. Not surprisingly, it found its way across the US-Mexico border and is a key ingredient in Tex-Mex dishes. Recipes of the Middle East, North Africa, India, Europe, Mexico and the American Southwest share in common this worldwide spice.

HOW TO USE

1. Use the pale green fruits or seeds whole or grind them into powder.

2. To make a cup of cumin tea, use one teaspoon of crushed seeds per cup of boiling water.

IN THE KITCHEN

Dry-frying cumin seeds for a few minutes before using them whole or grinding them helps to bring out the flavour.

'We use cumin, coriander, black pepper, cinnamon, parsley, mint, cloves. All are used as spices and herbs for cooking.' (Eastern KSA)

RECIPES

Falafel, p. 198
Couscous, p.195

DID YOU KNOW?

➴ In ancient Babylon, cumin was used in medicines to treat eye and ear problems, mouth disease, foot ailments and kidney stones.

➴ Cumin is an ingredient of the popular Saudi-Gulf spice mixture *baharat* (sometimes called Arabic spice or Middle East spice), which is used in lamb dishes and other Arabic recipes.

➴ Regular cumin should not be confused with black cumin (*Nigella sativa*), better known as black seed.

➴ The Roman historian Pliny reports that the ancients mixed crushed cumin fruits with water or bread for an all-purpose medicine. He also called cumin the best of all condiments, and he favoured the Ethiopian and African varieties.

➴ Al-Kindi, a leading physician of the Middle Ages, saw the value of cumin as a treatment for stomach ailments. He also included cumin in an oil for rheumatism of the knees and other joints.

FAMILY REMEDIES ACROSS ARABIA

Cumin relieves flatulence and bloating and stimulates the digestive process.

Childbirth: Fresh soup as a meal is good for the woman after delivery. It consists of fresh meat, chopped onion, and mixed spices of black pepper, turmeric and cumin. Boil these ingredients until meat is ready to eat. (Southern KSA) ᔕ Use fenugreek, *rashad*, black seeds, cumin, cinnamon, whole-wheat flour with honey and butter, meat and *thareed*, a dish with vegetables, tomato sauce and meat with small pieces of bread. (Central KSA) ᔕ For childbirth, use dates, *bukhoor* (incense) of *'ud*, cinnamon and cumin. (Eastern KSA) ᔕ To strengthen a mother after childbirth, use fenugreek, cress, black seeds, cumin, black pepper and ginger. (Northern KSA)

Colds or Coughs: Use Vicks cough syrup, boiled water with cumin, and a small spoon of sesame oil. (Western KSA)

Colic: Boil anise, cumin and peppermint (equal quantities) and add some crystalline sugar or honey. Then, put 7 drops of black seed oil and drink while hot and it is good for colic. (Eastern KSA) ᔕ Cumin and fennel are used to lessen abdominal pain, especially colic. (Southern KSA)

Diabetes: Mix 1 tablespoon of myrrh, 1 cup of *rashad*, $1/2$ cup black seed, $1/2$ cup ground pomegranate, 1 cup ground dried cabbage root and a teaspoon of cumin seeds. Eat on an empty stomach or with yoghurt to make it easier to eat. (Eastern KSA)

Flatulence (Intestinal Gas): Cumin and fennel are used to remove gases from the abdomen and to reduce colic. (Southern KSA)

Indigestion: Use ground cumin. (Southern KSA)

Liver Pain: Mix water with cumin and black pepper and drink it to reduce liver pain. (Southern KSA)

Menstrual Pain: For cramps, use cumin and boiled cloves with honey. (Central KSA)

Stomachache: Boiled cumin is sweetened and used for stomachaches and headaches. (Bahrain) ᔕ Use cinnamon, cumin and anise. (Southern KSA) ᔕ Use ginger and cumin. (Central KSA) ᔕ Use cumin and peppermint. Boil with water and drink. (Northern KSA) ᔕ For stomachaches, use cumin and myrrh. (Northern KSA)

RESEARCH

Cumin was one of seven edible plants shown in a Mexican university study to cause a significant reduction in blood sugar levels in healthy rabbits. (Roman-Ramos, R., et al. 'Anti-hyperglycemic effect of some edible plants.' *J Ethnopharmacol.* 1995 Aug 11; 48(1): 25-32.)

Cumin seeds and basil leaves fed separately to rats significantly decreased the incidence of two types of cancer cells in the rats' stomachs, according to a study at India's Cancer Institute. The researchers said the results indicate that cumin and basil 'may prove to be valuable anticarcinogenic agents.' (Aruna, K, and V.M. Sivaramakrishnan. 'Anticarcinogenic effects of some Indian plant products.' *Food Chem Toxicol.* 1992 Nov; 30(11): 953-6.)

DATES

Phoenix dactylifera
Arecaceae (Palm) Family
Arabic: *tamr*

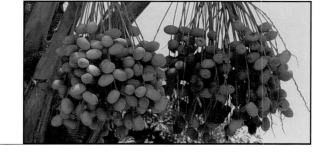

If any plant is a global symbol of Arabia, it is the date palm. Representations of *Phoenix dactylifera* appear on the national flag of Saudi Arabia as well as in many Arab corporate logos. The plant is so visibly prominent because of its historical importance to Arabian culture, economy and society. The Prophet Muhammad is reported to have said: 'There is among trees one that is pre-eminently blessed, as is the Muslim among men; it is the date palm.'

The date is the sweet, nutritious fruit of the date palm, a tall, hardy tree that thrives in arid regions. Saudi Arabia is home to some of the finest dates grown anywhere. The Kingdom produces about 870,000 tons of dates per year, representing some 15 per cent of total world production. More than 40 varieties of dates are produced in the Gulf region. According to common belief, the best of these – some say the best in the world – is called the *khalas*. Some 36 varieties, including the *khalas*, are cultivated in the al-Hasa oasis of the Eastern Province, one of the most extensive date farming areas in the world.

For centuries, the date fruit has provided the Bedouin with an energy-rich food that can be carried and stored easily in areas of hot, dry desert. The Bedouin eat dates with goat or camel milk to obtain protein, sugar, vitamins and minerals. While the date fruit provides nourishment and the leaves of the date palm are used for making ropes, cords and baskets, there is still yet another blessing offered by the palm. During and after pollination in the spring, the spathe (Arabic: *luqah*) – a leafy shield protecting the male or female flowers that grow from the date palm's single central bud – is often removed, boiled and distilled into a liquid that is used to treat stomach upsets.

HOW TO USE

1. Dates can be eaten fresh from the tree at varying stages of ripeness and sweetness, from yellow to reddish to brown in colour, or dried for storage.

2. For special treats, dates are sometimes pitted and stuffed with almonds or dipped in chocolate.

3. They are often chopped up and used in cooking.

4. Bedouins of the Eastern Province traditionally mixed pitted dates with milk and sheep fat for complete nutrition.

IN THE KITCHEN

Dates are the traditional food used to break the fast during the holy month of Ramadan. This versatile fruit is used in pastries, sweets, rice and vegetable dishes, and with meat, fish and fruit.

Date syrup is made by pressing dates with a heavy weight and then draining off the syrup. This syrup can be used in cooked dishes to help retain moisture and to add sweetness and flavour. It can also be eaten plain, or mixed with tahina (sesame seed paste) and spread on bread.

Clean dates by gently wiping with a damp cloth. Avoid exposure to too much moisture in order to prevent molding. When stored properly at room temperature, fresh dates keep for months. To prolong flavour and quality, fresh dates can also be refrigerated or frozen.

Ripe dates are traditionally dried in the sun and stored for use throughout the year. Dried dates store at room temperature (70°F/21°C) for up to 6 months and at lower temperatures (52°F/11°C) for considerably longer, from 3-4 years.

To rehydrate, pour boiling water over dried dates, using equal amounts of fruit and water, and soak for 15 minutes or to the desired texture. Alternatively, place dates in a steamer and steam to the desired texture.

DID YOU KNOW?

❧ The date palm was cultivated in ancient Mesopotamia and Egypt as early as 6,000 years ago. The Arabs brought the date tree to Spain, and Spaniards subsequently carried it to California and Arizona, where it thrives today.

❧ The palm tree requires watering only once every two weeks and is able to withstand the dry, hot days and cold nights of the harsh desert climate.

❧ A date palm at its peak may yield 300-400 pounds of fruit in a season.

❧ The date palm begins producing fruit when it is about seven years old and sustains abundant yields on average for 75 years, although the tree itself may live to be 150 years old.

❧ It takes about six or seven months for dates to ripen on the tree. The ripening process passes through four stages, from green to yellow to reddish to brown.

❧ Although only the female trees produce fruit, one male tree can produce enough pollen to pollinate 40-50 female trees. Pollen can be transmitted from male to female trees naturally, through wind and insects, or with human intervention.

❧ Dates are low in fat, cholesterol-free and high in carbohydrates, fibre, potassium and vitamins. Dates are 80% sugar. Remaining contents are protein and fat and mineral products, including copper, sulphur, iron, magnesium and fluoric acid.

❧ Five dates contain about 115 calories, nearly all from carbohydrates.

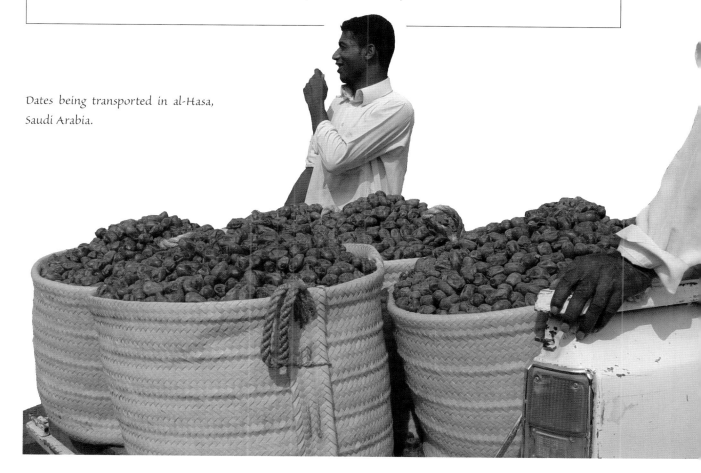

Dates being transported in al-Hasa, Saudi Arabia.

FAMILY REMEDIES ACROSS ARABIA

Saudi women have long chosen to eat dates when they are pregnant or nursing in order to make sure they are receiving adequate vitamins and to boost their energy.

In the Qur'an (19: 23-25), in labour with Jesus, Mary is guided to a palm tree to eat its dates and thereby lessen the pains of childbirth.

Appetite: If you lose your appetite, eat *halhul* (dates which have ripened on the tree) or drink *mesi* (dates crushed in water). (Socotra, Yemen)

Burns: In the past, we used dates mixed with a little salt, but nowadays we use medical ointments. (Central KSA)

Childbirth: For childbirth, eat lots of dates; drink cinnamon tea. (Bahrain) ❧ Eat dates and apply a mixture of olive and walnut oil to the stomach to make the delivery fast and easy. (Northern KSA) ❧ Eat yellow or brown dates before delivery. (Southern KSA) ❧ Use anise and dates. (Southern KSA) ❧ Use boiled cinnamon or cloves with honey and eat dates during labour. (Central KSA) ❧ Eat dates and massage with butter. (Central KSA) ❧ Eat seven dates and drink hot cinnamon (Central KSA) ❧ When you feel pain in the back, start eating as many dates as possible. This helps ease delivery. (Eastern KSA) ❧ Use dates, *bukhoor* of *oud*, cinnamon and cumin. (Eastern KSA) ❧ Use dates and cow's milk without sugar. (Eastern KSA) ❧ Use dates and cinnamon boiled in water. (Western KSA)

After Childbirth: For post-partum haemorrhage, drink *mesi* (dates crushed in water), for a week. Use the best variety of dates available. For retained placenta, drink *mesi* at regular intervals and keep on the move. (Socotra, Yemen) ❧ Drink a meat soup. Eat *aseeda*, or gruel, prepared with wheat flour (Southern KSA) ❧ To strengthen a mother after childbirth, use dates, black seeds, fenugreek and a plant called *al-faraa*. (Southern KSA) ❧ Use honey, yellow dates and soup, in addition to using myrrh and salt for washing. (Southern KSA) ❧ Use fenugreek with egg to strengthen the woman, prepared like custard and sweetened with sugar or date juice, molasses or dates. Also, eat gruel made from whole-wheat flour and sugar or date juice and sheep butter. (Eastern KSA) ❧ Eat gruel (whole-wheat flour with dates, butter and spices including black pepper) with fried egg in the morning. (Eastern KSA) ❧ Eat half-cooked liver and cow's milk. Also, eat *aseeda*. (Eastern KSA)

Cracked Bones: Mix black seed with dates and put on wound, covering with white wrapping, to treat cracks in bone (things a doctor can't reach). (Central KSA) ❧ Treat a broken hand by putting lamb's wool around the hand then placing palm sticks on top of it to serve as a splint. (UAE)

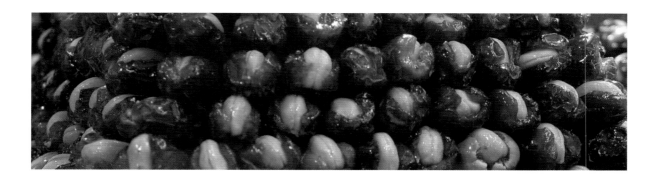

Diarrhoea, Phlegm and Bronchitis: Use dates to treat diarrhoea, phlegm and bronchitis by making a drink consisting of 50g. dates, 50g. raisins, and 50g. dried figs. Place in 1 litre of water and boil. (Eastern KSA) ❧ For diarrhoea, drink dates (from last year's pressed crop) crushed in water. (Socotra, Yemen)

Insect Bites: For the bite of a giant centipede, apply *mesi* (dates crushed in water) to the site. For a scorpion sting, drink *mesi*. (Socotra, Yemen)

Joint Pain: Mix dates with salt and heat. Wrap it with a towel and put it on the joints if you have pain. (Central KSA) ❧ There is a saying in Najd that 'dates are the nails for the knees,' meaning dates give knees strength. (Central KSA)

Nausea: Drink *mesi* (dates crushed in water). (Socotra, Yemen)

Newborn Care: Warm the pit of a date over coals, then wrap in a small handkerchief. Then put it on the area around the navel. (Southern KSA) ❧ Take a date seed, wrap it in clean cloth, then warm it over coals. Put it in the baby's navel and rub in all directions inside it. That helps the umbilical cord to fall very fast. (Southern KSA) ❧ Massage the navel with the pit of the date with myrrh and kohl. (Southern KSA)

Sore Throats: Use lemon, sesame oil and tahini with dates. (Eastern KSA)

Stomach Ailments: We buy *luqah* by the pint and add a teaspoonful to our tea, either instead of milk for taste, or as a medicinal compound for upset stomachs. (Eastern KSA) ❧ Use myrrh, *laban* and *luqah*. (Eastern KSA) ❧ For babies, use date water and/or flower water for stomachaches. (Central KSA) ❧ For babies, put dates in very warm water until water is brown. Give the liquid to the baby 2-3 times a day to treat stomachaches. (Eastern KSA) ❧ For babies, use sugar cane (natural sugar), date water, anise and fenugreek tea. (Central KSA)

RECIPES	Date cake, p. 199
	Date bars, p. 200
	Aseeda, p. 202

RESEARCH

A preliminary study at Kuwait University shows that date fruit possesses 'quite potent' antioxidant and antimutagenic properties, potentially useful in the fight against cancer. (Vayalil, P.K. 'Antioxidant and antimutagenic properties of aqueous extract of date fruit *(Phoenix dactylifera L. Arecaceae)*.' J Agric Food Chem. 2002 Jan 30; 50(3): 610-7.)

Dates contain fluorine, which helps protect teeth against decay. They contain selenium, believed to help prevent cancer and important in immune function. Dates also possess pectin, which may have important health benefits. A recent study describes dates as 'an almost ideal food, providing a wide range of essential nutrients and potential health benefits.' (Al-Shahib, W., and R.J. Marshall. 'The fruit of the date palm: its possible use as the best food for the future.' *Int J Food Sci Nutr.* 2003 Jul; 54(4): 247-59.)

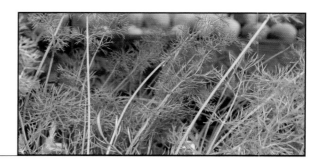

FENNEL

Foeniculum vulgare
Apiaceae/Umbelliferae (Parsley) Family
Arabic: *shamar, shumra, hulwa, habba helwa*

Fennel is an ancient Mediterranean herb with a variety of culinary and medicinal uses. The leaves and stalks of this feathery plant can be eaten as a vegetable – it is popular this way in Italy – but its dried fruits (sometimes called seeds) are more widely used in cuisines from Europe to China and beyond.

Since Babylonian times, fennel has often been confused with its cousin anise (*Pimpinella anisum*) and some Asian languages still do not distinguish between the two plants. But Arabs know the difference: anise is *anisun* and fennel is *shamar* or *hulwa*.

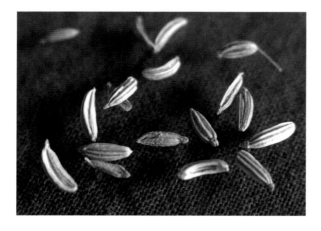

HOW TO USE

1. Chop the leaves or tender stems into soups or salads.

2. For tea, bring one cup of water to a boil. Pour over 1-2 teaspoons of crushed fennel fruits. Cover and steep for 10 minutes. Strain and drink in small cupfuls.

3. Chew the fruits to freshen the breath and allay hunger.

4. Grind seeds to powder for use in baking.

IN THE KITCHEN

The leaves of this plant have a pleasant aniseed scent and can be finely chopped and sprinkled on salads and cooked vegetables or used in soups and stews. Tender fennel stems may also be chopped into salads.

RECIPE

Baked Fennel with Goat's Cheese, p. 198

RESEARCH

Fennel greens were one of nine families of salad greens native to the Mediterranean that were found to have marked antioxidant properties. (El, S.N., and S. Karakaya. 'Radical scavenging and iron-chelating activities of some greens used as traditional dishes in Mediterranean diet.' *Int J Food Sci Nutr.* 2004 Feb; 55(1): 67-74.)

Fennel oil can decrease the intensity of infantile colic, according to a recent Russian study. (Alexandrovich, I., et al. 'The effect of fennel (*Foeniculum vulgare*) seed oil emulsion in infantile colic: a randomized, placebo-controlled study.' *Altern Ther Health Med.* 2003 Jul-Aug; 9(4): 58-61.)

FAMILY REMEDIES ACROSS ARABIA

Fennel is a well-known digestive aid. A tea of crushed fennel fruits is a natural remedy for flatulence, colic, or upset stomachs. The fennel fruit is antispasmodic, carminative, diuretic, expectorant and stimulant.

Colic: Boil the seeds with a little sugar for 10-15 minutes, then strain. When it is warm, give it to the baby. That helps to relieve swelling in the abdomen and to reduce colic. (Southern KSA) ⚘ Cumin and fennel are used to lessen abdominal pain, especially colic. Fennel is used a lot for breastfed children to reduce colic. (Southern KSA)

Flatulence (Intestinal Gas): Put fennel seeds in water and boil for 10-15 minutes. Then, strain the seeds and drink the liquid hot or cold. Fennel is also used ground with coffee or with dates. (Southern KSA)

Indigestion: Eat onion with date, fennel, black seed, thyme and cheese to aid indigestion. (Eastern KSA)

Rheumatism: You can add black seed to olive oil and fennel to treat rheumatism and pain in the joints. (Northern KSA)

Stomachache: Take cumin and fennel. (Southern KSA)

DID YOU KNOW?

⚘ Fennel is a member of the Apiaceae/Umbelliferae family and resembles its relatives dill and anise. It has lacy, feathery leaves and clusters of flowers that bloom a bright yellow.

⚘ Fennel was cultivated by the ancient Romans and remains popular in Italy to this day. Pliny the Elder, the Roman encyclopaedist, recommended fennel for 'dimness of vision'.

⚘ Florence fennel (F. v. azoricum), also known as finocchio, forms a bulb well-known in Italian cooking.

⚘ Medieval Arab physician al-Kindi prescribed fennel fruits, root, rind of root and extract for various remedies, including treatments for scrofula, moist ulcers, swelling, fever, stomach and liver pain, and for strengthening eyesight.

⚘ The Puritans combined fennel fruits with dill and caraway and carried them in little purses to prayer meetings. Chewing the seeds helped to quell hunger pangs.

⚘ Though of southern European origin, fennel is now a major herbal crop in India, China and Egypt.

⚘ Chinese traditional medicine prescribes fennel for abdominal pain, indigestion, hernias and food poisoning.

FENUGREEK
Trigonella foenum-graecum
Fabaceae (Legume) Family
Arabic: *hulba, hilba*

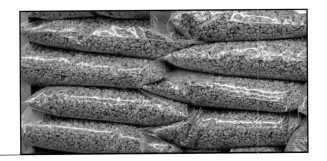

Fenugreek has grown in the Nile Valley since at least 1000 BC. Its brownish yellow seeds have long been used as a tonic and stomachic in the Arab countries and Iran.

In the Middle East today, it is still cultivated as a kitchen herb, a medicinal plant and as a food and fodder crop in Egypt, Yemen and in the Mediterranean region.

RESEARCH

Fenugreek is a major ingredient in a dietary supplement developed by Canadian researchers that resulted in significant weight loss in obese patients without raising the heart rate or blood pressure. (Woodgate, Derek E., and Julie A. Conquer, in *Current Therapeutical Research – Clinical and Experiment*, reported in *Biotech Week*, Aug. 13, 2003, p. 345.)

Studies have found that fenugreek helps improve blood sugar control in patients with insulin-dependent (type 1) and non-insulin-dependent (type 2) diabetes. (Sharma, R.D., et al. 'Effect of fenugreek seeds on blood glucose and serum lipids in type 1 diabetes.' *Eur J Clin Nutr* 1990; 44:301–6; Madar, Z., et al. 'Glucose-lowering effect of fenugreek in non-insulin dependent diabetics.' *Eur J Clin Nutr* 1988; 42:51–4.)

An extract of *Trigonella foenum-graecum* was shown in a recent study to have a significant inhibiting effect on the growth of human cancer (melanoma) cells. (Sathiyamoorthy, P., et al. 'Screening for Cytotoxic and Antimalarial Activities in Desert Plants of the Negev and Bedouin Market Plant Products.' *Pharm. Biology*, 1999, Vol. 37, No. 3, pp. 188-95.)

HOW TO USE

1. Cook the fresh green leaves like spinach.

2. Brew the dried leaves as a tea.

3. Sprout the seeds to add a light curry flavour to salads or sandwiches.

4. Use either the leaves or powdered seeds for medicinal poultices.

5. Soak seeds overnight to create a gelatinous substance for making pastes.

6. Boil the seeds in water. Add a teaspoon of the boiled seeds to food or drinks

7. Infuse ground seeds in water to make a tea.

IN THE KITCHEN

The spicy flavours of Yemen include fenugreek-based mixtures served with bread and used as dip. Flour mixed with ground fenugreek makes a tasty bread. Fenugreek seeds are an ingredient of *halawa* or *halva*, a sesame-based Middle Eastern sweet.

Add ground seeds in moderation to flavour food or mix with other spices to create homemade curries. Dry-fry seeds before grinding. A light roast yields a mellow flavor. A darker roast will result in a more bitter taste.

RECIPES

Sprouted Fenugreek Seeds, p. 186
Yemeni Fenugreek Paste, p. 203

FAMILY REMEDIES ACROSS ARABIA

Fenugreek is valued for a variety of reasons. As one resident of central Saudi Arabia explains, 'Fenugreek softens the throat, the chest and the abdomen. It is also good for flatulence, phlegm, haemorrhoids and to stimulate menstruation. When you shampoo with it, it makes your hair curly. Some people say that if people knew its benefits, they'd value it like gold.'

In Abha and other parts of the Asir (southwestern Saudi Arabia), fenugreek tea is used to treat rheumatoid arthritis and other bone and joint disorders, according to Noura bint Muhammad al-Saud and her co-authors in the book *Abha*: *Bilad Asir*. Fenugreek is also used as a remedy for intestinal ailments, colic and diarrhoea.

Fenugreek seeds contain approximately 30 per cent mucilage, a slippery substance used as a natural emollient.

Bleeding: For external cuts or wounds, use *aqit*, a strong dried yoghurt, ground to powder and put on the wound, or use fenugreek or *shabba*. Apply each one separately. (Northern KSA)

Bones: Fenugreek strengthens bones and joints. It's also good for fractures. Add ground seeds to food as treatment. (Central KSA)

Breast Abscesses and Mastitis: Grind fenugreek seeds to a powder, add water and apply the paste to the painful area. (Socotra, Yemen)

Childbirth: Fenugreek, *rashad* (cress) and black pepper are good for 40 days after delivery. (Central KSA) ❧ Black seed is used with honey, cress and fenugreek. Together they are used as a medication for stomachaches and after giving birth. Take twice a day. (Eastern KSA) ❧ After childbirth, fenugreek helps to strengthen the back and return the uterus to its natural position. (Southern KSA) ❧ Boil the seeds and drink to stimulate milk flow. (Southern KSA) ❧ Use *julab*, a herb drink that should be taken regularly for 40 days, myrrh, and fenugreek to strengthen a mother after childbirth. (Western KSA) ❧ To strengthen a mother after childbirth, use chicken or meat soup with vegetables and fenugreek. (Western KSA) ❧ Use fenugreek, anise, black seeds and wheat to strengthen the mother. (Western KSA) ❧ To strengthen a new mother, mix 5 egg yolks, 2 teaspoons honey, 2 tablespoons butter, and 1/3 cup fenugreek. (Eastern KSA) ❧ Use fenugreek with egg to strengthen the mother. It is made like custard sweetened with sugar or date juice (molasses). (Eastern KSA) ❧ To strengthen a mother, cook fenugreek with *marquq*. (Eastern, Central and Northern KSA) ❧ For childbirth, use boiled fenugreek and *mahaleb*. (Northern KSA) ❧ To strengthen a mother after childbirth, use fenugreek, black pepper and wild ghee (clarified butter). (Northern KSA)

Diabetes: Soak one tablespoon of seeds overnight in a glass of water and drink each morning. (Yemen) ❧ Grind fenugreek seeds into powder. Mix one teaspoonful with water and drink to lower blood sugar levels. (KSA)

Headaches: In the past, people used olive oil, cloves, henna and fenugreek. Heat on stove and put on the area of the pain. (Northern KSA)

Liver: Fenugreek is used to treat liver problems. (UAE)

(continued overleaf)

FAMILY REMEDIES ACROSS ARABIA

Menstrual Cramps: Use fenugreek and cinnamon. (Western KSA) ❧ Drink a cup of boiled fenugreek sweetened with honey in the morning and evening. Also, put a few drops of black seed oil in every hot drink. (Eastern KSA) ❧ For menstrual cramps, use peppermint and fenugreek. (Eastern KSA) ❧ For menstrual cramps, use myrrh and fenugreek. (Northern KSA)

Newborn Care: Herbs used for babies include caraway, fenugreek, anise, water and sugar. (Eastern KSA) ❧ Put fenugreek and henna on the weak area on the top of the baby's head. (Northern KSA)

Stomachaches: For stomachaches, use fenugreek, cress, cinnamon, peppermint and sage. Or, you can drink onion juice mixed with boiled fenugreek and sweetened with honey or crystalline sugar. Drink once a day to remove gases and colic. (Eastern KSA) ❧ For babies, use anise, black seeds and fenugreek. (Southern KSA)

DID YOU KNOW?

❧ The Latin name *foenum graecum* means 'Greek hay.' The dried leaves and seeds of fenugreek are said to smell like hay.

❧ The food industry uses the ground seeds and essential oil of fenugreek to produce imitation maple flavouring.

❧ Greek botanist Dioscorides, who lived in the first century AD, recommended oil of fenugreek to soften mature abscesses and hard lumps around the uterus, to treat burns and chilblains, and to eliminate dandruff.

❧ In selecting fenugreek for medicinal use, Dioscorides recommended careful selection of fenugreek: 'Choose that which is new, scours the hands, is bittersweet in taste and does not smell too much like fenugreek, for that is the best.'

❧ The Arab physician al-Kindi used Syrian fenugreek in a dressing to dissolve cysts, in an electuary for cold-related phlegm and rheumatism, and in an herbal bath for victims of incontinence.

❧ Fenugreek is generally quite safe, but the seeds can stimulate the uterus and may cause miscarriages, so they should not be used during pregnancy, warns University of Arizona botanical medicine specialist Francis J. Brinker.

❧ Palestinian folk medicine prescribes fenugreek for treating menorrhagia, postpartum bleeding and cramps, GI gastro-intestinal tract inflammation, and distention, as well as for increasing the amount and flow of breast milk.

❧ The ancient Egyptians used fenugreek in the mummification process.

❧ Fenugreek gives off what many today consider an objectionable smell when consumed. The smell is released with perspiration and clings to one's clothes.

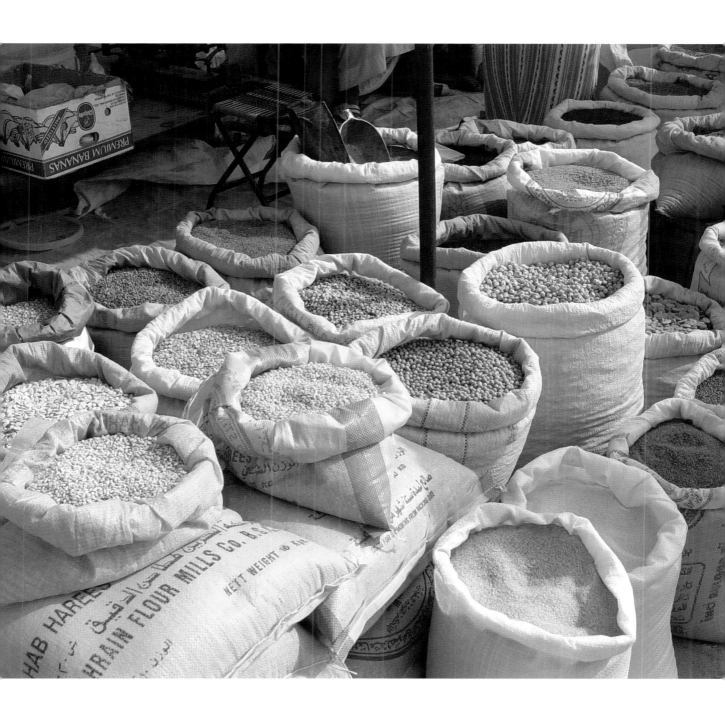

An outdoor market at Qatif, Saudi Arabia.

FRANKINCENSE

Boswellia sacra or *B. carteri* or *B. thurifera*
Burseraceae (Frankincense and Myrrh) Family
Arabic: *luban*
Other English: Olibanum, Oil of Lebanon

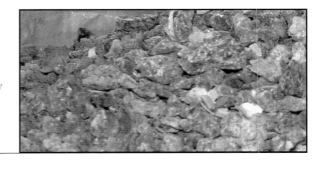

Frankincense is crystallized tree sap – a hardened gum or resin exuded by a small tree that grows in the coastal regions of the southern Arabian Peninsula and nearby coastal East Africa. In ancient times, frankincense was a precious commodity, sometimes more valuable than gold. Merchants brought this treasure to the great civilization centres of Europe and Western Asia by sea journey and by a land trail through Yemen and up the Arabian Red Sea coast to the Levant. The pharaohs of Egypt used it for perfume, medicine and embalming the dead. Clumps of incense were discovered among the treasures buried in the tomb of Tutankhamen, who died in 1339 BC.

The Hebrew prophet Moses, who led the exodus from Egypt in the 13th century BC, used pure frankincense as one of the ingredients of a perfume to be used in the Tabernacle (Exodus 30:34) and pure myrrh as one ingredient of a holy anointing oil (Exodus 30:23-25).

Frankincense has been burned for centuries during royal and religious rites, lending dignity to ceremonies of many faiths and symbolizing the ascent of prayers to God. In Saudi Arabia and other Gulf countries, frankincense is used as incense today, though not in religious ceremonies. Its uses focus on personal hygiene and health.

Although the frankincense gathering season lasts from May through mid-September, the product is available year-round in traditional local markets of the Middle East.

Due to unique climatic conditions, the best frankincense is produced by trees growing in the mountainous Dhofar region of Oman. Frankincense is also grown in Yemen, Ethiopia, Somalia and India.

HOW TO USE

1. Chew as a gum. This is a popular use, as frankincense has a mild, pleasant taste and helps to eliminate bad breath. The juice derived from the gum is thought to benefit the kidneys and liver.

2. Suck on a granule to relieve nausea.

3. Soak frankincense granules in water and drink the strained liquid.

4. Burn as incense for a pleasant scent or waft on clothing.

IN THE KITCHEN

It is not uncommon in Arabia for families to keep a glass jar of frankincense or myrrh covered with water in the refrigerator. Then, when a remedy is called for, the liquid is strained and ready to consume.

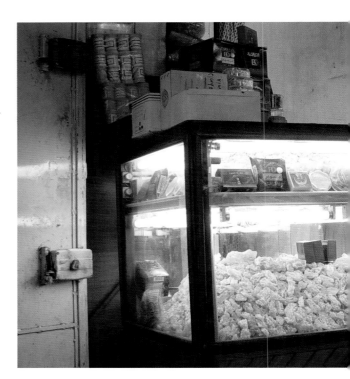

DID YOU KNOW?

🦢 Frankincense comes in five main colours: white, pale lemon, pale amber, pale green and dark amber. The colour of the gum resin is influenced by its harvest time. A whiter gum is collected closer to autumn, whereas a darker colour is harvested closer to spring.

🦢 The ancient Hebrews imported Boswellia trees before the Babylonian Exile (586-538 BC) to furnish incense for use in certain rituals. After the Second Temple was destroyed by the Romans (70 AD), the use of incense disappeared from Jewish worship.

🦢 Frankincense was one of three gifts that the Magi presented to the infant Jesus (Matthew 2:11). The others, of course, were gold and myrrh.

🦢 Tenth-century Persian physician Ibn Sina (also called Avicenna) used frankincense in treatments for tumours, ulcers, vomiting, dysentery and fever.

🦢 Frankincense today remains an ingredient in various incense mixtures burned in rituals of the Roman Catholic and Orthodox churches.

🦢 Western herbalists regard frankincense essential oil as an anti-inflammatory, antiseptic and astringent, and say it is useful as a uterine tonic during pregnancy and labour.

🦢 Charred frankincense has been used to make kohl, the black powder traditionally used by women in the Middle East to paint their eyelids.

A frankincense stall in Old Town Jeddah, Saudi Arabia.

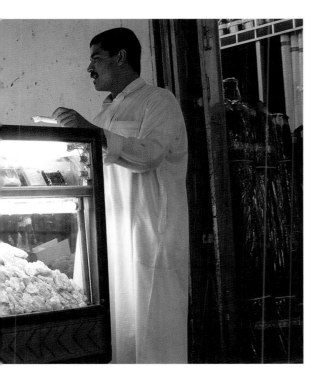

RESEARCH

Boswellic acids found in frankincense have shown 'promising results' in clinical trials in treating certain chronic inflammatory diseases, including rheumatoid arthritis, chronic colitis, ulcerative colitis, Crohn's disease, bronchial asthma and peritumoral brain edemas. (Ammon, H.P. '[Boswellic acids (components of frankincense) as the active principle in treatment of chronic inflammatory diseases].' *Wien Med Wochenschr.* 2002;152(15-16):373-8.)

One type of boswellic acid, acetyl-11-keto-beta-boswellic acid (AKBA), has been shown to be toxic to certain human tumour cells. (Park, Y.S., et al. 'Cytotoxic action of acetyl-11-keto-beta-boswellic acid (AKBA) on meningioma cells.' *Planta Med.* 2002 May;68(5):397-401.)

FAMILY REMEDIES ACROSS ARABIA

Luban dhakar ('male frankincense' – light-coloured, globular) is used for medicinal purposes. It relieves sore throats and coughs and is also considered good for the stomach. *Luban dhakar* is not usually chewed as gum because it is bitter and tastes unpleasant. It also crumbles into small pieces and lacks the consistency of gum.

Bleeding and Swelling: Frankincense is heated and its smoke is used to heal wounds and swollen areas. (Eastern KSA)

Childbirth: Following delivery of a baby, some women remove their clothes and stand over a smoke of burning frankincense, onion skins, black seed and *shabba* (alum). The warmth is said to ease pain from the contracting uterus. (KSA) ❧ To strengthen a mother after childbirth, use modern medicines, honey, *maraq* and frankincense. (Western KSA)

Coughs: Frankincense is useful for chests and relieves coughs. You take it like myrrh. (Central KSA) ❧ Frankincense we drink soaked with a little myrrh and cress for coughs. And we rub the chest with olive oil with a little Vicks. (Central KSA) ❧ We use frankincense to treat coughs and colds. Soak frankincense granules in warm water, let the mixture sit for three hours, then drink the liquid. (Eastern KSA) ❧ Take honey with lemon, bitter frankincense and ginger. (Western KSA)

Diabetes: I use bitter frankincense to treat diabetes and help indigestion. (Eastern KSA) ❧ Also we use frankincense and myrrh for those with diabetes and hypertension because it reduces high sugar levels in the blood. (Eastern KSA)

Diarrhoea: Use myrrh, frankincense and tea. (Eastern KSA)

Liver: The juice derived from the gum is thought to benefit the kidneys and liver. (KSA)

Lungs: Boiled frankincense with water and honey is useful because it strengthens and activates the lungs and is good for treating hydrocephalus (abnormal accumulation of fluid in the brain). (Eastern KSA) ❧ Boil frankincense in water and drink it. It's good for the chest. (UAE)

Memory: Frankincense sharpens the memory and reduces coughing. (Northern KSA) ❧ It helps clear the brain. (Yemen)

Nausea: Frankincense is used by pregnant women in the first month to help eliminate nausea. Suck it in your mouth. (Eastern KSA)

Odours: Frankincense strengthens cheek muscles, prevents stomach gas, and soaks up odours in the air. If you chew it often, it even eliminates, or soaks up, the smell of sweat. (Eastern KSA) ❧ Burned with *bukhoor* (incense), frankincense soaks up odours from the air. (Eastern KSA)

Oral Care: We use frankincense to clean the mouth and exercise jaw muscles and to treat colic in the abdomen. (Eastern KSA) ❧ Chew Shehri frankincense (almost white in colour) for healthy teeth and gums. (Yemen) ❧ Frankincense: there are two kinds. Use Shehri frankincense as *bukhoor*. Use Lami frankincense as a gum. (Central KSA)

Stomach Complaints: Frankincense is for stomach pain. (Northern KSA) ⚘ Use frankincense for coughs and indigestion. (Central KSA) ⚘ I use frankincense because it is useful for colic, indigestion, constipation, halitosis and coughs. (Eastern KSA) ⚘ Boil amber-coloured powdered frankincense to make an infusion for an upset stomach. (Yemen)

Saudi Aramco Nursery, Dhahran, Saudi Arabia.

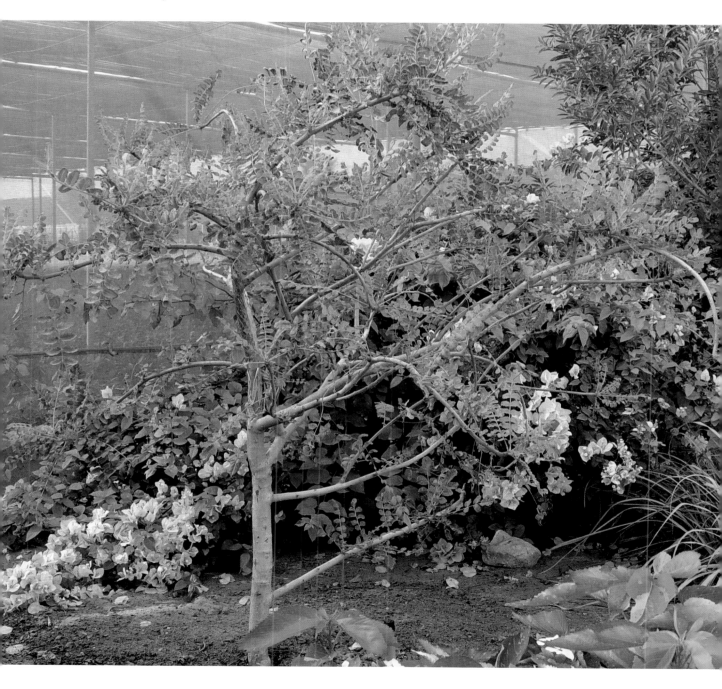

GARLIC
Allium sativum
Alliaceae (Onion) Family
Arabic: *thum*

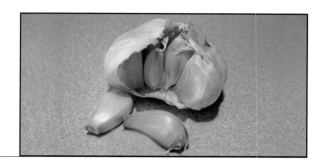

Botanist David Hooper, studying plants in Iran and Iraq in the 1930s, observed that garlic was the potherb *par excellence* of the East – not only was it used in a dizzying array of culinary dishes, but it also aided digestion and was a gastric stimulant. If anything, Hooper's comment was an understatement. We now know garlic has a wealth of other medicinal properties to complement its enduring value as a cooking herb.

Garlic, a bulbous perennial, probably originated in Central Asia, the only place where it grows wild. There are plants in other lands referred to as 'wild garlic', which are part of the Allium genus but not true garlic (*A. sativum*).

Garlic has edible flowers but it is primarily grown for its bulbs, each of which contains 12-20 cloves. Garlic has been cultivated by mankind from time immemorial. Hundreds of varieties have emanated from Asia across the globe.

HOW TO USE

1. Crush, chop or use garlic cloves whole to flavour dishes.

2. Bake, roast or grill a bulb of garlic. When softened, squeeze out the pulp from the individual cloves to eat.

3. Mash the softened pulp of baked garlic to form a smooth paste and use it in soups, sauces, and dips. Alternatively, grind fresh garlic to a paste with a mortar and pestle.

IN THE KITCHEN

When frying, use enough olive oil or butter to coat the pan and stir often. Garlic burns quickly if cooked over high heat.

Store garlic in a cool, dark pantry. Garlic stored in the refrigerator quickly dries out and rots.

| RECIPES | Roasted Garlic, p. 196 | Baba Ghannouj, p. 205 | Hummus, p. 206 |

RESEARCH

Garlic has been recognized for its medicinal properties for thousands of years, but scientific research into how it works is relatively recent. Investigations have been conducted over the past decade into garlic's antibacterial, antiviral, antifungal and antiprotozoal properties. *Allium sativum* has also been shown to have beneficial effects on the cardiovascular and immune systems. (Harris, J.C., et al. 'Antimicrobial properties of *Allium sativum* (garlic).' *Appl Microbiol Biotechnol.* 2001 Oct; 57(3): 282-6.)

Garlic has been studied extensively for its potential anti-cancer properties. One analysis of 18 such studies found that six cloves of raw or cooked garlic a week had a significant effect in preventing colorectal and stomach cancer (Fleischauer, Aaron T., et al. 'Garlic consumption and cancer prevention: meta-analyses of colorectal and stomach cancers.' *American Journal of Clinical Nutrition*, Vol. 72, No. 4, 1047-52, October 2000.)

FAMILY REMEDIES ACROSS ARABIA

Bites and Stings: Use garlic for ant bites. (Northern KSA) ⚘ Use a clove of garlic to relieve the pain of a bee sting. (UAE) ⚘ Rub a raw garlic clove on the spot where a scorpion stings you, and it will heal. (Eastern KSA)

Childbirth: Use fenugreek, cress, cinnamon, sage, peppermint as well as old traditional foods like gruel and dates, meat sauce, Hasawi rice (red rice from al-Hasa) and garlic. (Eastern KSA)

Colds or Coughs: Swallow one clove of garlic with a glass of milk every day. (Western KSA)

Bleeding: Put an ointment made of ground garlic on the wound even if it hurts, since this prevents gangrene, which can lead to amputation of the limb. Also, you can clean wounds by mixing ground garlic in warm water and cleaning the wound with it to kill the microbes. (Eastern KSA)

Diarrhoea: Eat yoghurt with garlic. (Western KSA)

Fatigue: Eat garlic with food. (Central KSA)

Hair Loss: Use garlic, *jarjeer* (arugula) oil, sesame oil and black seed oil. (Southern KSA) ⚘ Use garlic, lemon and jarjeer. (Central KSA) ⚘ Use henna, garlic, coconut oil, sesame, castor oil and aloe. (Central KSA) ⚘ To treat hair loss, use henna, egg, *sidr*, olive oil, aloe vera, *jarjeer* juice, parsley and garlic. (Eastern KSA) ⚘ Use a mix of oils: onion juice, almond oil, sesame and garlic. Apply *jarjeer* oil and henna on hair with hibiscus. (Eastern KSA)

Heart Trouble: Garlic, onion and exercise. (Central KSA) ⚘ Put mashed garlic in oil and leave covered out in the sunlight for 40 days. Then eat one spoonful every day for 40 days to treat narrowing of arteries due to fat deposits and hypertension. (Eastern KSA)

Stomachache: Take honey and black seed, or garlic and vinegar. (Southern KSA) ⚘ Drink pear juice mixed with three garlic cloves before you go to sleep each day. When you have colic, rub the abdomen with garlic oil mixed with olive oil. (Eastern KSA)

Vomiting: To stop vomiting, cut a clove of garlic or onion, sniff it and eat it raw. (Socotra, Yemen)

Warts: My grandmother used garlic to prevent warts from reappearing, and to kill warts. (Bahrain)

DID YOU KNOW?

❧ According to tradition, the Prophet Muhammad recommended garlic, applied topically, to remedy viper bites and scorpion stings.

❧ Garlic was a principal ingredient in 'Four Thieves Vinegar', used as protection against the plague at Marseilles in 1722. Legend recounts that four thieves confessed to using liberal amounts of this aromatic vinegar during the plague and were thus able to plunder the dead bodies of its victims without fear.

❧ Despite garlic's known antibiotic activity, and despite Internet rumours to the contrary, there have been no scientific studies showing garlic has any effect against anthrax.

GERMANDER

Teucrium polium
Lamiaceae (Mint) Family
Arabic: *ja'dah* or *ja'ad, bu'aythiran*
Other English: Poley, Golden Germander,
Felty Germander

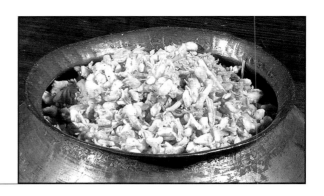

Early in the 20th century, Bedouins of Northern Arabia used dried leaves of the germander plant as an insect repellant to protect the leather portions of stored armour, according to Czech anthropologist and explorer Alois Musil (1868-1944). Saudi Bedouins today report that the dried leaves of this plant are smoked in a pipe to treat rheumatism. Its leaves are also said to cure fevers, such as malaria and cholera.

Germander is one of three species of Arabian plants sometimes locally called *bu'aythiran*. The other two are *Achillea fragrantissima* (yarrow) and *Artemisia judaica* (Biblical or Judean wormwood).

A perennial shrub found not only in Arabia but also in the hills and deserts of the Mediterranean region, *Teucrium polium* has long been in folk medicine to treat diabetes, inflammations, ulcers, high blood pressure and other ailments.

HOW TO USE

1. Dry the leaves.

2. Smoke the dried leaves.

3. Infuse its small woolly flowers, mixed with its stalks and leaves, to make a tea.

IN THE KITCHEN

To preserve the quality of dried leaves and flowers, store in an airtight container, out of direct light, and in a cool location. Glass jars keep excess air and moisture out and are the best choice for maintaining the integrity of an herb for the longest period of time.

DID YOU KNOW?

🔖 There are approximately 100 species of *Teucrium*. General distribution includes Egypt, Palestine, Turkey, Iraq, Saudi Arabia, Bahrain and Iran.

🔖 Arab traditional medicine, according to ethnobotanist James A. Duke, prescribes *Teucrium polium* for abscesses, abdominal pain, childbirth, insect bites, jaundice and malarial fever.

🔖 In Southern Iran, an aqueous extract of the dried aerial parts of *Teucrium polium* is used by Type 2 diabetic patients as an anti-diabetic drug.

FAMILY REMEDIES ACROSS ARABIA

Germander is considered a vermifuge, stimulant and tonic.

Diabetes and Rheumatism: *Ja'ad* leaves have been used for diabetes and rheumatism. (Northern KSA)

Oedema: *Ja'ad* reduces the amount of liquids in the body. (Central KSA)

Purgative: An infusion concocted from the leaves has been used as a purgative. (Bahrain)

Stomach and Intestinal Troubles: An infusion of the tender parts of germander is used for stomach and intestinal troubles. (KSA)

RESEARCH

Iranian researchers have warned that use of *Teucrium polium* should be discouraged as an herbal remedy because of potential toxic effects on the liver as well as the reported ineffectiveness of commonly used doses on blood sugar levels of diabetic patients. (Ansari Asl, A., et al. 'The Effect of Extract of *Teucrium Polium* on Blood Sugar and Insulin Levels of Type 2 Diabetic Patients.' *Shiraz E-Medical Journal*, March and April 2002, Vol. 3, No. 2.)

In southern Iran, experimental trials have shown that high doses of *Teucrium polium* can decrease blood sugar in streptozocine-induced diabetic animals. (Suleiman, M.S., et al. 'Effect of Teucrium Polium boiled leaf extract on intestinal motility and blood pressure.' *J Ethnopharmacol.* 1988; 22: 111-116; Ghahharzadeh, A. 'Antidiabetic effects of extract of Teucrium polium on diabetic rats, dissertation (in Persian).' *Kerman University of Medical Sciences* 1996; 45-47; Zal, F. 'Antidiabetic effects of an aqueous extract of Teucrium polium on streptozocine induced diabetic rats, (in Persian).' Thesis, *Shiraz University of Medical Sciences*, 2001; 38-9.)

Greek researchers have reported significant anti-oxidant activity in ethanol extracts of *Teucrium polium* and nine other members of *Lamiaceae*. (Couladis, M., et al. 'Screening of some Greek aromatic plants for antioxidant activity.' *Phytother Res.* 2003 Feb; 17(2): 194-5.)

Teucrium polium was one of the leading antimalarial agents identified among 66 desert plant extracts tested on cultures of *Plasmodium falciparum*. (Sathiyamoorthy, P., et al. 'Screening for Cytotoxic and Antimalarial Activities in Desert Plants of the Negev and Bedouin Market Plant Products.' *Pharmaceutical Biology.* Jul 99, Vol. 37, Issue 3, p. 188-95.)

The dried extract of *T. polium*, at specific dosages over prolonged periods, are reported to have induced liver and kidney trouble in rats (Khleifat, Khaled, et al. 'The Chronic Effects of *Teucrium polium* on Some Blood Parameters and Histopathology of Liver and Kidney in the Rat.' *Turk. J. Biol.*, 26, (2002), 65-71.)

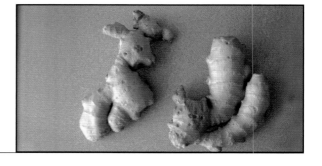

GINGER
Zingiber officinale
Zingiberaceae (Ginger) Family
Arabic: *zanjabil, zanjabil sini*
Other English: Chinese Ginger

Ginger root – actually a rhizome – is popular in a wide variety of cuisines. Chefs of Southeast Asia, China, Japan and Korea typically use ginger in its fresh state. Many recipes and spice blends in the Middle East call for the use of dried ginger.

Ginger is available fresh, dried, crystallized, ground, pickled and preserved as stem ginger (fresh, young ginger shoots which have been peeled, sliced, cooked and finally preserved in sugar syrup). Ginger is well preserved in syrup and sugar, and it was in this form that much of the ginger carried in ginger jars along the ancient spice routes was transported.

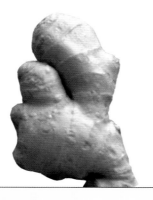

HOW TO USE

1. Finely chop, grate or grind to a paste fresh ginger for use in sauces, soups and stir-fries.

2. Use a press to extract juice from finely chopped or grated fresh ginger. Collect the juice for use in sauces, marinades and salad dressings.

3. Grind dried ginger to powder.

IN THE KITCHEN

If cooking with hard, dried pieces of ginger, bruise the ginger first with the bottom of a jar to crush and open the fibers to release the flavour.

Unpeeled fresh ginger may be kept up to four weeks in the refrigerator if well wrapped in plastic wrap. If the ginger becomes dry, soft and wrinkly, it is time to throw it out.

Ginger tea with honey or with honey and lemon is normally served during the winter.

RESEARCH

Ginger extract inhibits the growth of *Helicobacter pylori*, a microorganism believed to cause dyspepsia, peptic ulcer disease and the development of gastric and colon cancer. (Mahady, G.B., et al. 'Ginger (Zingiber officinale Roscoe) and the gingerols inhibit the growth of Cag A+ strains of Helicobacter pylori.' *Anticancer Res.* 2003 Sep-Oct; 23(5A): 3699-702.)

Ginger appears to be an effective treatment for nausea and vomiting in pregnancy, according to recent studies. (Sripramote, M., and N. Lekhyananda. 'A randomized comparison of ginger and vitamin B6 in the treatment of nausea and vomiting of pregnancy.' *J Med Assoc Thai.* 2003 Sep; 86(9): 846-53; Portnoi, G., et al. 'Prospective comparative study of the safety and effectiveness of ginger for the treatment of nausea and vomiting in pregnancy.' *Am J Obstet Gynecol.* 2003 Nov; 189(5): 1374-7.)

FAMILY REMEDIES ACROSS ARABIA

Ginger increases circulation and acts as a diaphoretic to produce perspiration. Both of these actions help to speed the removal of toxins from the body.

Childbirth: Rub stomach of pregnant woman with oil and ginger and oil of walnut to be ready for delivery of child. (Central KSA) ﷼ To strengthen a new mother, use fenugreek, cress, black seeds, cumin, black pepper and ginger. (Northern KSA)

Cholesterol: Ginger is used to reduce the amount of cholesterol in the blood. (Central KSA)

Colds and Coughs: To treat a head cold, insert some ground ginger in the nostrils. (Socotra, Yemen) ﷼ Use ginger for colds and influenza. (Eastern and Southern KSA) ﷼ Ginger helps digestion. It's useful for the stomach and it destroys phlegm and is useful for colds. Boil ginger with saffron and sugar and drink it as tea. (Central KSA) ﷼ Boil ginger with water and sugar to treat colds. (Southern KSA) ﷼ Combine black seed, cardamom, ginger and olive oil. Heat on the fire. After that, rub on skin and body. Make tea with ginger and drink it hot. (Northern KSA) ﷼ Use peppermint and ginger with milk. (Northern KSA) ﷼ For colds or coughs, use honey with lemon, bitter frankincense and ginger. (Western KSA) ﷼ For colds or coughs, take ginger and black pepper in milk and soup. (Central KSA) ﷼ Use ginger and lemon and honey for coughs and colds. (Central KSA) ﷼ Use milk with ginger for coughs or colds. (UAE)

Congestion: Fresh ginger beaten or crushed and eaten to remove phlegm or sputum. (Southern KSA)

Diarrhoea: Use ginger and yogurt and bitter tea (strong/dark). (Central KSA)

Eyes: To treat a small abscess in the rim or inner corner of the eye, pierce the abscess and make it bleed, then chew a piece of dried ginger and apply the paste to the abscess. (Socotra, Yemen)

Headaches: Use peppermint, saffron, ginger and water (drink). (Southern KSA) ﷼ Ground ginger and ground sugar. Swallow them (one spoon). Then follow it with a glass of water. (Northern KSA)

Menstrual Pain: For cramps, use boiled cinnamon with a little sugar as wanted and a little ground ginger. (Southern KSA) ﷼ Cinnamon and ginger. Boil together for 25 minutes, then drink. (Central KSA) ﷼ Drink a tea of boiled cinnamon, ginger and mint. (Northern KSA)

Sore Throats: Use ginger, cress and myrrh. (Central KSA) ﷼ Green ginger with lime and honey. Boil in water and drink. (Northern KSA)

Stomachache: Use ginger and cumin. (Central KSA)

DID YOU KNOW?

◈ The ginger plant probably originated in China. About half the world's crop is now produced in India.

◈ The Chinese have used ginger for centuries to treat stomachaches, digestive disorders, nausea, rheumatism and poor circulation.

◈ Confucius, the well-known philosopher who lived twenty-four centuries ago, used ginger as a staple in his diet.

◈ Externally, ginger may be used in a fomentation to treat stiff joints and inflammations. In addition, the juice of fresh grated ginger mixed with equal parts of sesame or olive oil may be massaged into the skin to relieve muscle pain. This same oil may be applied to the head to relieve headaches.

◈ Headaches have also been relieved by heating a piece of fresh ginger, slicing several thin pieces, and applying the slices to the affected area. Cooled slices should be replaced with warm slices.

◈ Constituents contained in ginger stimulate the production of digestive fluids which help to break down food and prevent fermentation and the formation of gas. Ginger has earned the description 'carminative,' or that which removes gas from the alimentary canal.

◈ Al-Kindi, the 9th-century physician, used Chinese ginger in a collyrium to improve vision and in medications for sore throat, earache, arthritis and stomach upset.

◈ Another ginger species, wild ginger (*Zingiber zerumbat* or *Curcuma zerumbat,* Arabic: *zurunbad*) is exported from India to some parts of the Middle East. It is used like Chinese ginger as a condiment and an ingredient in traditional medicine. Al-Kindi recommended wild ginger in a treatment for nosebleeds.

RECIPE

Ginger Tea with Honey and Lemon, p. 181

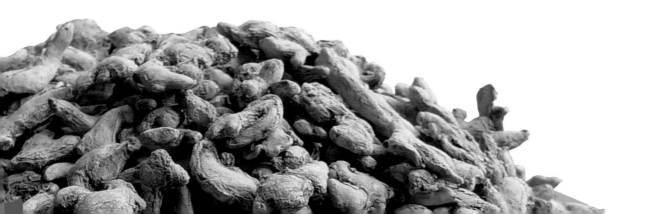

HASAWI RICE

Oryza sativa
Poaceae (Grass) Family
Arabic: *ruzz hasawi*
Other English: al-Hasa Red Rice

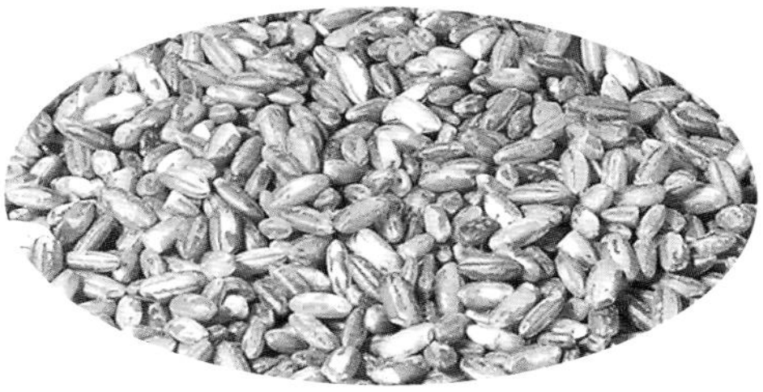

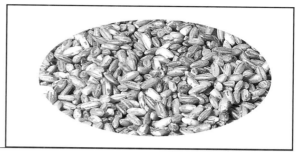

Hasawi rice was once grown fairly extensively in the al-Hasa oasis of eastern Saudi Arabia, but today is harder to find. The underground water resources used for irrigation in al-Hasa – an area of the world famous for its extensive date palm orchards – are scarcer and much more carefully husbanded nowadays than in the past.

In the 1960s, Saudi Arabia reported its Hasawi rice production to the UN Food and Agriculture Organization. Al-Hasa was then known as the world's driest rice-producing region. But by the 1990s, the FAO was no longer keeping track of Saudi rice statistics – the quantities were too small to record.

In the old days, much of al-Hasa's red rice crop would be sold to Bedouins, who could not afford the more expensive white rices from India and other parts of Asia. Today, Hasawi rice is a rare and expensive delicacy. Long known to be rich in nutrients, Hasawi rice is particularly prized by new mothers and others seeking to regain their health or strength.

RECIPE *Hasawi Rice with Shrimp, p. 197*

FAMILY REMEDIES ACROSS ARABIA

Childbirth: After giving birth, a mother regains her strength by eating Hasawi rice. (Eastern KSA)

HOW TO USE

Hasawi rice is washed in cold water, cooked in boiling water and eaten as part of a meal.

IN THE KITCHEN

Hasawi red rice, like brown rice, takes longer to cook than conventional white rice. In al-Hasa, it is often seasoned with locally popular spice blends.

DID YOU KNOW?

- Red rice is only partially milled and, like brown rice, retains the colour of its bran coating.
- True red rice, like Himalayan red and al-Hasa red, should not be confused with 'red yeast rice,' a Chinese rice that has been treated with red yeast *(Monascus purpureus)* and is used for medicinal purposes, particularly cholesterol control.
- In the 1930s, rice was cultivated north of al-Hasa 'over immense areas' of southern Iraq, according to botanist Evan Guest. The rice, cultivated as a summer crop in the marshes and flow canals, was hulled after harvest and called timan. A small amount of rice farming continues in southern Iraq to this day.
- The Persian physician Najib al-Din al-Samarqandi (died 1222 AD) recommended *Oryza sativa* as a treatment for dysentery.

RESEARCH

Rice bran – the remaining hull on red or brown rice – has shown promising disease-preventing and health-related benefits, according to recent research. Diseases that may respond to rice-bran treatment include cancer, hyperlipidemia, fatty liver, hypercalciuria, kidney stones and heart disease. (Jariwalla, R.J. 'Rice-bran products: phytonutrients with potential applications in preventive and clinical medicine.' *Drugs Exp Clin Res.* 2001;27(1):17-26.)

HENNA

Lawsonia inermis or L. alba
Lythraceae (Loosestrife or Pomegranate) Family
Arabic: *hinna*

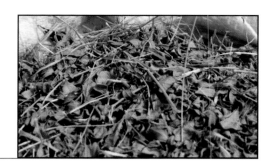

Yasmeen is excited but nervous. In two days she will marry Ali and her life will change completely. Tonight she is enjoying her henna party, a traditional gathering for women before the wedding day. Yasmeen reclines on cushions as a henna specialist decorates her hands and feet with intricate brownish-orange designs. Her guests entertain her with songs and dances. While the henna on her hands is drying, her friends feed her sweetmeats and hot sweet tea. Life is wonderful!

Dried henna leaves ground into powder form the basis of this important cosmetic dye valued by women throughout the Middle East. The dye is widely used to decorate hands and feet and to colour hair. Recipes vary, as different families might add tea water, coffee, hibiscus, lime juice or other ingredients to adjust colour, shade and quality.

HOW TO USE

1. Dry the leaves.

2. Grind leaves into powder.

3. Mix powdered henna with water and any other desired ingredients to form a paste. Then, apply to the body for cosmetic or medicinal purposes.

IN THE KITCHEN

Use a stain-resistant bowl when mixing up henna paste.

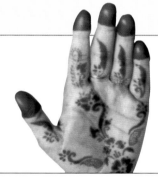

DID YOU KNOW?

☙ Since the days of the Prophet Muhammad, elderly men in Arabia have sometimes used henna to dye their beards.

☙ Residents of Qatif and al-Hasa have been known to decorate their white donkeys with henna.

☙ Much of the henna in Saudi Arabia's Eastern Province is imported from India, according to botanist James P. Mandaville. But henna from al-Madinah is also sold in Eastern Province markets, and is highly prized.

☙ Herbalist Jethro Kloss cites henna as a remedy for headaches and, in tea form, as a gargle for sore throats.

☙ Medical anthropologist John Heinerman has recommended the use of henna paste for herpetic lesions and sores afflicting AIDS patients.

☙ King Solomon compared his love to a henna flower: *'My beloved is to me a cluster of henna blossoms in the vineyards of En-gedi.'* (Song of Solomon 1:14)

FAMILY REMEDIES ACROSS ARABIA

Henna is put on the soft spot of a newborn's head and is also used to treat burns, headaches and hair loss. In addition, it is used with salt and cress for cuts and combined with black seed and vinegar to treat pus-producing infections. Henna is also used as a pain reliever.

Burns: Use henna to treat burns, cuts and mouth sores. (Central KSA) ❧ Use henna for burns. (UAE)

Chicken Pox: Families once used henna for children with chicken pox. (Central KSA)

Colds and Fevers: Put henna on the bottom of the feet to treat colds and fevers, especially for children. (Central KSA)

Cuts: For cuts, apply henna, cress and salt. (Central KSA) ❧ Henna and black seed mixed with vinegar are useful for cuts and pus-producing infections. (Central KSA)

Foot Pain: Henna is for beauty, or to help with foot pain. Mix ground henna with a little water until it becomes like a dough. Spread it on the soles of the feet. Also, you can mix henna and water into a runny mixture and put it on the hair. This nourishes hair roots and scalp. (Southern KSA) ❧ Henna is a treatment for cracks in the heel of the foot, and for relief of foot pain, treatment of dandruff, as well as for dyeing hair, strengthening it, and treating split ends. (Eastern KSA)

Hair Loss: Use cloves, salt and henna mixed together every two weeks or once a month. (Northern KSA) ❧ Use castor oil and henna. (Northern KSA) ❧ To prevent hair loss, use cress and henna. (Central KSA) ❧ I use henna and olive oil. (Central KSA) ❧ For hair loss, use henna, egg, *sidr*, olive oil, aloe vera, *jarjeer* juice, parsley and garlic. (Eastern KSA) ❧ Use a mix of oils, onion juice, almond oil, sesame and garlic. Put *jarjeer* oil and henna on the hair with hibiscus. (Eastern KSA)

Headache: Henna helps to reduce headaches, head pain and foot pain. (Southern KSA) ❧ Put henna on hair and scalp to control headaches. (Central KSA) ❧ In the past, olive oil, cloves, henna and fenugreek were used for headaches. Mix, heat on the stove and put on the head. (Northern KSA) ❧ Use henna, olive oil and *mahaleb*. (Eastern KSA)

Infections: Henna is mixed with butter and used to treat tumours, scabies and infections with pus. It also prevents cold sores and boils that appear suddenly on the legs. (Central KSA) ❧ It's used as a disinfectant for wounds and as a remedy for foot pain. (Eastern KSA)

Measles: Henna is for beautification and for treatment of measles. (Southern KSA)

Summer Heat: Use henna to moisten the scalp and cool the head in hot weather. (Southern KSA) In summers, use henna to cool the head. It is also applied to burns to help in healing. (Eastern KSA)

RESEARCH

An extract of powdered henna leaf was found to be the most effective of 20 Yemeni herbal medicines in countering bacterial growth. (Ali, N.A., et al. 'Screening of Yemeni medicinal plants for antibacterial and cytotoxic activities.' *J Ethnopharmacol.* 2001 Feb ; 74(2): 173-9.)

Henna leaves are known to be strongly toxic against fungi, largely because of the presence of an antifungal compound known as Lawsone. (Tripathi, R.D., et al. 'A fungitoxic principle from the leaves of *lawsonia inermis lam.' Experientia.* 1978 Jan 15; 34(1): 51-2.)

HERBAL WATERS

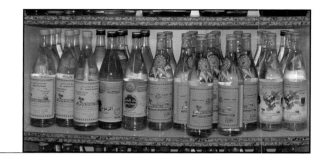

Lining some supermarket shelves in Bahrain, Saudi Arabia, the United Arab Emirates and other Middle Eastern countries are bottles of a highly regarded remedy called herbal waters. These beneficial waters have been distilled from the leaves, bark, roots, pods and flowers of medicinal herbs cultivated and collected locally or purchased from countries abroad, such as India or Lebanon.

Herbal waters are comprised of one main ingredient but may also include a herbal mixture added to achieve optimal effectiveness in treating a particular ailment. These herbal formulas are closely guarded by their manufacturers. No sugar or carbonation is added.

These aromatic waters include rose hip, palm pollen, *luqah* (date-palm spathe), nettle, fennel, cumin and cinnamon bark, to name a few.

HOW TO USE

Many of the herbal water bottles include labels listing the beneficial properties of the water and dosage information in English. Follow instructions carefully.

IN THE KITCHEN

Herbal waters are valued as flavourings for other liquids. Drink herbal waters plain or dilute in other beverages.

DID YOU KNOW?

🐾 Herbal waters are the by-product of the steam distillation of plant material for the production of essential oils. They are filled with water-soluble nutrients that are part of the plants' immune systems. Their properties are similar to those of essential oils.

🐾 Herbal waters, also known as hydrosols or hydrolates, have been distilled and used in India and the Middle East for many hundreds of years. Recently they have become more widely known in the West, primarily as a part of aromatherapy.

🐾 Throughout the centuries, orange blossom water has been used as a liver equalizer and heart tonic.

🐾 Rose water has been used in the Middle East since ancient times to flavour a variety of sweets and desserts, including baklava.

FAMILY REMEDIES ACROSS ARABIA

Herbal waters are reputed to treat disorders ranging from indigestion to heart disease. Local consumers swear by their healing powers:

Darseen (**cinnamon**) **water** helps treat lower-respiratory diseases and revitalizes the stomach.

Al-Heaj **water** relieves rheumatism, infections of the urinary tract and bladder, kidney and liver pain, and jaundice.

Al-Helwa (**fennel**) **water** aids digestion, quenches the thirst and serves as a tranquillizer for children.

Hindeban (**chicory**) **water** is used as a tonic for the heart, kidney, liver and stomach, serves as a diuretic and lowers cholesterol.

Karafs (**celery**) **water** is taken for kidney and urinary function.

Kozaboon **water** purifies the blood, lowers body temperature, counters allergies, and serves as a diuretic and tonic.

Luqah **water** is known as a heart tonic, is refreshing and thirst-quenching, and helps reduce vomiting. The male palm tree produces *luqah*, a medicinal drink. It is good for stomach problems. (Eastern KSA)

Margadoosh (**sweet marjoram**) **water** relieves flatulence, counters constipation and acts as a digestive and diuretic. *Margadoosh* (sweet marjoram) is used to treat indigestion. (Eastern KSA)

Na'naa' (**Mint**) **water** aids digestion, relieves constipation and stomach pain, serves as a tranquillizer and flavours tea and juice.

Shatirra **water** is regarded as a blood purifier and a remedy for liver and skin diseases like itching.

Sukkari **water** is known to regulate blood sugar levels.

Zaytoon (**olive**) **water** is used to treat high blood pressure.

Zamooteh **water** is said to eliminate stomach pain and liver pain, as well as intestinal gas.

RESEARCH

See specific herbs.

HIBISCUS

Hibiscus sabdariffa
Malvaceae Family
Arabic: *karkady, karkaday*
Other English: Indian Sorrel, Jamaican
Sorrel, Java Jute, Red Sorrel, Roselle,
Rozelle, Sorrel

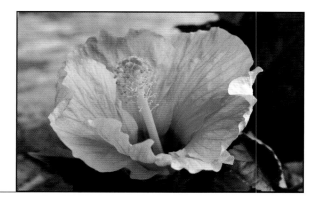

In the remote deserts of Upper Egypt and farther south in Sudan's central province of Kordofan, Karkaday plantation workers harvest the seed-pods of *Hibiscus sabdariffa*. By hand, they strip off the bright red calyces enveloping the pods and lay them out to dry in the sun for three to four days. The maroon, almost purple-black *karkaday* is then ready for the marketplace – at home and abroad.

Karkaday sold in the markets of the Arabian Peninsula is commonly imported from Egypt, the Sudan, Syria and Jordan.

HOW TO USE

1. Dried calyces are boiled to make a red tea.

2. Freshly picked calyces may be chopped and added to fruit or lettuce salads.

3. The young leaves and tender stems can be eaten raw in salads or cooked as greens.

4. In Africa, the seeds (although somewhat bitter) have been ground to a meal and used for food and have also been roasted as a substitute for coffee.

IN THE KITCHEN

A popular drink in the Middle East is the tart, bright red hibiscus tea, derived from boiling the dried red calyces. The tea is sweetened with sugar and can be served hot or iced.

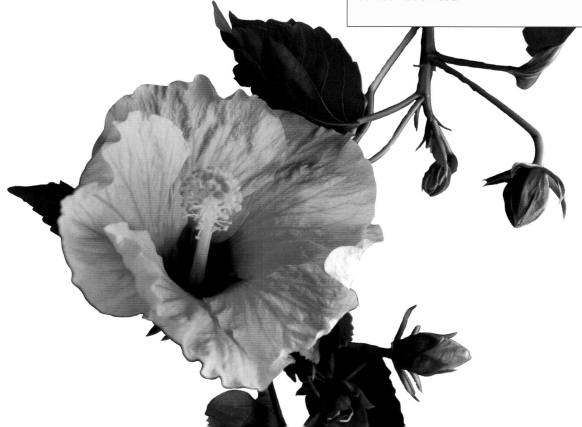

FAMILY REMEDIES ACROSS ARABIA

Hair Loss: Use a mix of oils, onion juice, almond oil, sesame and garlic. Put *jarjeer* oil and henna on hair with hibiscus. (Eastern KSA)

High Blood Pressure: Drink hibiscus tea to decrease blood pressure, but it affects the teeth if it is used too much. (Central KSA)

Kidneys: Hibiscus is useful for the kidneys. (Central KSA)

RESEARCH

Hibiscus tea has been shown to lower blood pressure. (Haji Faraji, M. and A.H. Haji Tarkhani. 'The effect of sour tea *(Hibiscus sabdariffa)* on essential hypertension.' J *Ethnopharmacol.* 1999 Jun; 65(3):231-6.)

Dried flower extracts of *Hibiscus sabdariffa* have demonstrated protective antioxidant effects in laboratory rats. (Tseng, T.H., et al. 'Protective effects of dried flower extracts of *Hibiscus sabdariffa L.* against oxidative stress in rat primary hepatocyctes.' *Food Chem Toxicol.* 1997 Dec; 35(12):1159-64.)

DID YOU KNOW?

⁖ The entire hibiscus plant (leaves, seeds, calyces and roots) is edible.

⁖ It is generally believed that African slaves first brought hibiscus seeds to the New World.

⁖ In Pakistan, hibiscus calyces have been recommended as a source of pectin for the fruit-preserving industry because they possess 3.19% pectin.

⁖ Hibiscus seeds are employed as an aphrodisiac in Mayanmar (Burma) and as a laxative in Taiwan. The seeds are also regarded as excellent feed for chickens.

⁖ In East Africa, the brownish-yellow hibiscus seed oil is claimed to heal sores on camels. Also in East Africa, the calyx infusion, called 'Sudan tea,' is taken to relieve coughs, and hibiscus juice is mixed with salt, pepper, asafoetida and molasses, and taken as a remedy for biliousness.

⁖ Infusions of hibiscus leaves or calyces are considered diuretic, cholerectic, febrifugal and hypotensive in the folk medicine of India, Africa and Mexico. The infusion is also thought to decrease the viscosity of the blood and stimulate intestinal peristalsis.

⁖ In Brazil, the bitter roots are considered to have stomachic, emollient and resolutive properties. In the Philippines, the roots are roasted, skinned and eaten to stimulate appetite.

⁖ Senegal supplies much of the hibiscus used to make extracts for flavouring liqueurs or as a natural colouring agent for drinks, foods, and meats. The dried calyces are squeezed into great balls weighing 175 lbs (80 kg) in preparation for shipment to pharmaceutical and food manufacturers in Europe.

HONEY

Arabic: *asal*

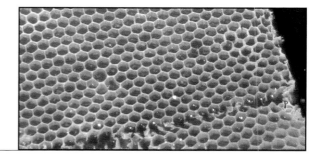

Saudi Arabia produces relatively little honey, but the average Saudi family consumes about a kilo of honey per month. So it is no surprise that Saudi merchants travel to Yemen and Oman to purchase very expensive and highly prized honey, rich in flavour and in medicinal qualities. The most frequent buyers come from Saudi Arabia, Bahrain and Kuwait.

Explorer Wilfred Thesiger reported that men from the Qarra region of southern Oman travelled with him and 'carried butter, firewood, and a pot of wild honey which they would sell in the market'. Today, wild honey is still collected from warm-climate dwarf Asiatic bees *(Apis florae)* in Dhofar and along the southern coast of Oman.

A more remote source of honey is the Wadi Du'an, a valley in Yemen just south of the Rub al-Khali, where beekeeping traditions date back at least a millennium. This area is also famous for its bee sellers, who establish a market along the main road each March to sell hives and swarms of bees.

Honeys differ in colour and flavour depending on the region they are from and which flowers the bees feed on. A favourite type of honey is that produced by bees fed on the *sidr* tree *(Zizyphus spina-christi)*.

HOW TO USE

1. Eat a teaspoon of honey plain or mixed with other healthful substances, such as black seed.

2. Add honey to teas and other liquids as a sweetener.

3. Use honey as a substitute for sugar.

4. Dip warm bread into a mixture of honey and clarified butter, and sprinkle with black seeds.

5. Cut into a honeycomb-like cake and eat it with your fingers.

IN THE KITCHEN

Yemeni honey shop proprietor Islam Ahmed Ba Dhib, quoted in *Aramco World* (January-February 1995), describes a traditional way to preserve meat in honey: 'Cut up either sheep or goat meat and submerge it in honey for six months. You must be careful to use a ceramic or glass container. It is a dish that rich people eat for breakfast or at weddings.'

RESEARCH

In addition to its antibiotic properties, honey has been shown to promote scar-free healing in some cavity wounds by limiting the production of collagen. (Topham, J. 'Why do some cavity wounds treated with honey or sugar paste heal without scarring?' *Woundcare Journal*, Vol. 11, No. 2, February 2002.)

Egyptian researchers have shown that honey and black seed *(Nigella sativa)* work together to halt certain types of cancer growth in rats. (Mabrouk, G.M., et al. 'Inhibition of methylnitrosourea (MNU) induced oxidative stress and carcinogenesis by orally administered bee honey and Nigella grains in Sprague Dawely rats.' *J Exp Clin Cancer Res.* 2002 Sep; 21(3): 341-6.)

FAMILY REMEDIES ACROSS ARABIA

Many black seed remedies (*see* Black Seed) call for the use of honey. Cooked honey is said to be ineffective as a medicine.

Burns: Rub a mixture of equal amounts of honey and Vaseline on the burn twice a day until the burned skin scales. Or use a mixture of an egg and a spoonful of honey and put on the burn. Put melon core on the skin to treat sunburn. (Eastern KSA) ✿ Apply honey and cold milk. (Southern KSA) ✿ Use honey and cold water. (Central KSA)

Childbirth: Honey is a perfect medicine to help women regain strength after childbirth. (Yemen) ✿ Regular doses of honey may help produce a male heir. (Yemen) ✿ Strengthen a mother with dates, honey, boiled cinnamon, ghee, black seed and *al-lawz al-bajl* [green almonds]. (Western KSA) ✿ Use honey with lemon, bitter frankincense and ginger. (Western KSA) ✿ Eat honey and dates. (Southern KSA) ✿ To strengthen a mother, use milk and a spoonful of honey. Mix together and drink. (Central KSA) ✿ Drink honey in the beginning of labour (a *finjan*, or Arabic coffee cup) to facilitate delivery and use honey also as a vaginal douche by mixing warm water with honey. (Eastern KSA) ✿ To strengthen a mother after childbirth, let her drink a mixture of 5 egg yolks, 2 teaspoons honey, 2 tablespoons butter and 1/3 cup fenugreek. (Eastern KSA)

Colds and Coughs: Use lime with tea and honey. Swallow one clove of garlic with a glass of milk every day. (Western KSA) ✿ Take *za'tar* (thyme) with hot water, myrrh and honey. (Western KSA) ✿ Drink ginger tea with lemon and honey. (Central KSA) ✿ Use pure honey with lemon juice and sesame oil, twice a day. (Central KSA) ✿ Take 2 tablespoons of honey and dissolve in water, boiling until you have vapour and inhale it through the mouth. Gargle honey dissolved in water with some salt. Also, put chopped onion in a cup of honey and leave it for 3 hours; then strain the honey and take a spoonful after a meal – it's good for both adults and children. (Eastern KSA) ✿ Use honey with lemon for coughs or colds. (UAE). ✿ Use honey with turmeric for colds or coughs. (UAE)

Cuts and Wounds: To treat infections, take a *finjan* of honey and a *finjan* of whale liver oil and mix them. Rub on the wound after cleaning it with an antiseptic which is honey in warm water. Then, put a bandage on every day and drink a lot of honey every day (1 *finjan*). (Eastern KSA) ✿ To treat infection on external cuts and wounds, apply honey and cold milk. (Southern KSA) ✿ Use honey or salt on external cuts or wounds. (UAE)

Fatigue: Use 1 spoonful of honey everyday as an antibiotic. Also, strain boiled walnut leaves sweetened with honey and drink as tea every day. Also, drink onion juice mixed with tomato juice and some salt to strengthen the body anytime. Also, grind radish seeds in onion juice with powdered thyme and eat with olive oil and cheese to strengthen the body. (Eastern KSA)

General Health: Take a spoonful of honey every morning. (Central KSA) ✿ A spoonful of honey a day helps elderly men stay young. (Yemen)

Continued on p.89

DID YOU KNOW?

☙ Flowers provide bees with pollen (containing fats, proteins, vitamins, and minerals) and nectar (containing sugar, a source of energy), which they use as food. Bees make honey from the nectar.

☙ Honey contains more than 25 different sugars, each of which has a different effect on the human metabolism.

☙ For many reasons, bacteria do not survive well in honey, so it is one of the very few foodstuffs that does not spoil.

☙ Honey is mentioned as a food of the Sumerians in the *Gilgamesh* epic, dating back to about 3,000 BC.

☙ The ancient Egyptians used honey to fight infection in open wounds.

☙ Jacob sent honey, along with balm, spices, myrrh, nuts and almonds, as gifts to Egypt in order to secure the release of his captive sons. (Genesis 43:11)

☙ Avicenna, the 11th-century physician who wrote the *Canon of Medicine*, regarded honey as an aphrodisiac. His view was widely shared in the Arab world, and remains popular today. This perception is not just Middle Eastern: honey is also considered an aphrodisiac in Japan.

☙ Honey is not only the sweetener of choice, but is considered by Avicenna to be 'the food of foods, the drink of drinks and the drug of drugs'. The best-known of Avicenna's herbal formulas, called *jawarish*, are ground, sifted and preserved in a honey base.

☙ Doctors stopped using honey as a wound dressing when antibiotic treatments were developed in the 1940s. Today, with the growth of bacterial strains resistant to antibiotics, new attention is being focused on this ancient remedy.

☙ Honey is a delivery medium for many Ayurvedic drugs.

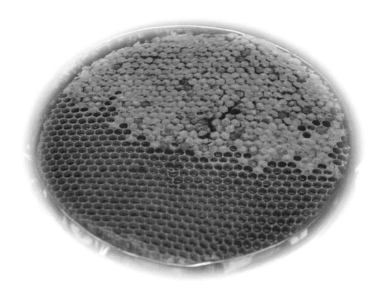

FAMILY REMEDIES ACROSS ARABIA (*cont.*)

Heart Trouble: Drink cold water sweetened with 2 tablespoons of honey every day on an empty stomach when a person has inflammation of the cardiac muscle or Parkinson's disease. (Eastern KSA)

Indigestion: We use soaked peppermint and soaked basil. Also, boil an unpeeled onion, then remove the peel and mash in honey and eat in a sandwich. Also, eat onion with dates, fennel, black seed, thyme and cheese for indigestion. (Eastern KSA) ❧ Take honey and black seed. (Southern KSA)

Insomnia: Use a tablespoon of black seed mixed with a cup of hot milk, sweetened with honey, and drink before sleeping. Also, drink a cup of warm milk sweetened with honey and drink it one hour before you sleep, which helps you to have a deep sleep. (Eastern KSA) ❧ The best way to treat insomnia is this mixture: 3 small spoons of vinegar, 1 *finjan* of honey. Put this mixture in a glass container and take some of it every evening at sleeping time (2 small spoonfuls). If it doesn't work after thirty minutes, try 2 more spoonfuls after an hour. This is much better than sedatives. (Eastern KSA) ❧ For trouble sleeping, take milk and honey or chamomile. (Northern KSA)

Intestinal Worms: Use *marbahey*, a hot honey, to get rid of intestinal worms. It is to be avoided by pregnant women, however, because it can cause miscarriage. (Yemen)

Sore Throats: Use orange, lemon and honey. (Southern KSA) ❧ Take green ginger with lime and honey. Boil in water and drink. (Northern KSA) ❧ Use 1 spoonful of honey in ¹/₂ cup water and mix, then gargle three times a day. Also, drink soaked peppermint. Also, put a hot onion compress around the neck and above the larynx. Gargle with onion juice and honey three times a day. (Eastern KSA) ❧ Soothe sore throats with honey. (UAE)

Stomachache: Use honey and dried pomegranate peelings. (Northern KSA) ❧ For the baby, use anise in water and honey in water for stomachaches. (Eastern KSA)

The beekeeper's area at Bin Bakr Farm, Taif, Saudi Arabia.

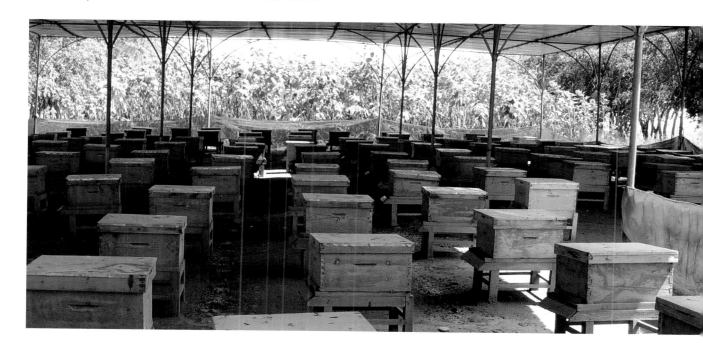

INCENSE

Arabic: *bukhoor*

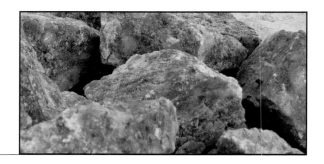

For centuries, incense – aromatic smoke – has been used for medicinal purposes. From about 4,000 BC many ancient texts on medicines, perfumes and incense mention frankincense and myrrh. In Arabia, these popular aromatics are still used to promote healing, either individually or in combination with other natural substances. Cinnamon, sandalwood, mastika, black seed, cumin, cardamom, perfume oils and the scented tropical wood known as '*ud* (aloeswood or agarwood, *Aquilaria malaccensis*) are also part of this healing tradition. Specific mixtures of these and other fragrant substances result in a variety of wonderful incense aromas and are often closely-held family or commercial secrets. *Bukhoor* mixtures can have as many as 10 or more ingredients.

These aromatics are burned to produce a pleasant odour and to welcome guests. Popular at weddings and social events,

HOW TO USE

Burn ingredient(s) on hot coals, usually in an incense burner, and fan the smoke into clothes, hair or area of the body requiring its medicinal or fragrant qualities.

IN THE KITCHEN

While mostly used in other rooms of the house, *bukhoor* is sometimes used in the kitchen. A family from Najran reports placing sugar on coals or ground coffee on the stovetop to create a nice smell in the kitchen, especially after cooking fish.

incense is wafted through rooms before, during and sometimes after special occasions. Guests are honoured when given incense with which to fan their clothing, underarms and hair. In the past, incense was offered when guests were ready to leave, not before. Men use incense before going to Friday prayers at the mosque.

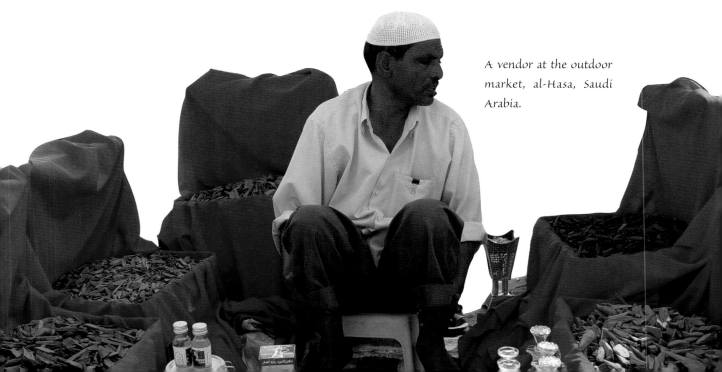

A vendor at the outdoor market, al-Hasa, Saudi Arabia.

FAMILY REMEDIES ACROSS ARABIA

To receive the benefits of *bukhoor*, the patient often stands over or near an incense burner as it releases fragrant smoke, bringing the *bukhoor* to the affected area.

Childbirth : Use *bukhoor* of *'ud*, cinnamon and cumin. (Eastern KSA) ✿ Burn *bukhoor* with coal and waft into the painful area. (Eastern KSA) ✿ Combine *laban thakr* (male frankincense), crushed myrrh, black seed and crushed *shabba* (alum) and burn as *bukhoor*. Use twice a day for 10 minutes to aid recovery from childbirth. (Eastern KSA) ✿ Use *bukhoor* of myrrh and *shabba* after childbirth to heal the wound/surgery. Do this twice a day, morning and afternoon. Said one Saudi woman: 'My aunt delivered a baby and was healed after two weeks using myrrh and *shabba*, while it usually takes one month to recover.' (Southern KSA)

Flatulence (Intestinal Gas): For gas or stomachache (resulting from change of temperature, for example) burn *bukhoor* of *'ud* under you for 20 minutes. (Eastern KSA)

Odours: Use Shehri frankincense (the highest quality, from the mountains of Dhofar, Oman) as *bukhoor*. (Central KSA) ✿ Use black seed as *bukhoor* along with another substance added to produce a pleasant smell. (Northern KSA) ✿ Burned with *bukhoor*, myrrh (as well as *mastika*) soaks up odours from the air. (Eastern KSA)

Menstrual Pain: My grandmother used to use *bukhoor* of myrrh for dysmenorrhoea. Apply cool to the vagina. (Eastern KSA)

DID YOU KNOW?

✿ Saudi males often scent their gutras (headcloths) and *thobes* (robes) with *'ud*.

✿ *Bukhoor wilada,* available in local markets, is a ready-made *bukhoor* mix intended for use following childbirth. It contains, among other ingredients, *mastika* and *'ud*.

✿ Some Saudi families maintain the custom of carrying a newborn baby around the house with a *mabkhara* (incense burner) during the first 10-15 days of life.

RESEARCH

Scientists in Germany have been studying Boswellic acids – the active ingredient in incense – for their role in treating chronic inflammations. (Ammon, H.P.'[Boswellic acids (the active agent in incense) for the treatment of chronic inflammatory diseases]'. *Med. Monatsschr. Pharm.* 2003 Sep; 26(9): 309-15.)

Scientists in Denmark have studied risk factors for chronic obstructed lung disease among women in Saudi Arabia. They found *no evidence* that incense burners contributed to such disease. Instead, a major risk for Saudi women was found to be exposure to indoor open wood fires for periods of 20 years or more. (Dossing, M., et al. 'Risk factors for chronic obstructive lung disease in Saudi Arabia.' *Respir. Med.* 1994 Aug; 88(7): 519-22.)

LAVENDER

Lavandula dentata
Lamiaceae (Mint) Family
Arabic: *khuzama*
Other English: French Lavender, Fringed
Lavender

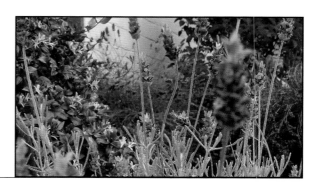

Lavender has been used for culinary and medicinal purposes since ancient times. Its medicinal legacy lives on in parts of the Middle East. In 1937, botanist David Hooper reported that flower heads of a species of lavender (*Lavandula dentata*) were being sold in Tehran, brought from Shiraz. He described this type of lavender as an ancient drug used by the Greeks and referred to by Arabian and Persian physicians.

L. dentata is one of the more widely distributed lavenders in the wild. Travellers to the mountainous region of Western Arabia find it growing as a common shrub. According to A.G. Miller of the Royal Botanic Garden in Edinburgh, it is found in Arabia (Saudi Arabia, Yemen), North Africa (Algeria and Morocco), South and Central Spain, and the Balearic Islands. White, lavender and pink flowered forms are found in Arabia and North Africa.

HOW TO USE

Use fresh or dried lavender flowers to make tea.

IN THE KITCHEN

Steeping lavender blossoms in boiled water yields lavender tea. It may be sipped plain or spiced with aromatic herbs like rosemary, thyme, cloves, cinnamon or whatever is in your spice cupboard. Around the world today, lavender flowers flavour foods such as cookies, cakes, breads, lemonade and sugar.

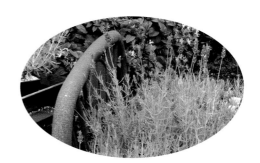

RESEARCH

Iranian researchers have confirmed the effectiveness of one species of lavender (*L. angustifolia*, English lavender) as a folk remedy in the treatment of painful and inflammatory conditions. (Hajhashemi, V., et al. 'Anti-inflammatory and analgesic properties of the leaf extracts and essential oil of *Lavandula angustifolia* Mill.' J Ethnopharmacol. 2003 Nov;89(1):67-71.)

L. dentata and some other species of lavender have properties that lower blood sugar, according to researchers. (Gamez, M.J., et al. 'Hypoglycemic activity in various species of the genus Lavandula. Part 2: *Lavandula dentata* and *Lavandula latifolia*.' Pharmazie. 1988 Jun;43(6):441-2.)

FAMILY REMEDIES ACROSS ARABIA

Flatulence (Intestinal Gas): Thyme, lavender and willow are used as a remedy for gases. (Northern KSA)

Urinary Problems: In the southern Hijaz and other nearby areas, an infusion of *L. dentata* flowers, taken first thing in the morning and before going to bed, is recommended for urine retention and for dissolving kidney or ureter stones. (Southern KSA)

DID YOU KNOW?

❧ Lavender infusions are used for compresses, applied to the forehead for headaches, wrapped around aching joints, and applied to relieve sinus congestion as well as tiredness and tension.

❧ In Iran, lavender infusions are used to treat catarrh and malaria. They are also used for washing wounds and skin eruptions.

❧ The essential oil of lavender is used for burns, insect bites and to encourage a restful night's sleep.

❧ Arab physicians of the Middle Ages used lavender as an expectorant and an antispasmodic.

❧ In the eastern and northern Arabian Peninsula, the Arabic word for lavender, *khuzama*, is applied to another plant species with fragrant purple flowers, *Horwoodia dicksoniae*. Species from the true lavender genus, Lavandula, are more commonly found in western and southern Arabia.

❧ Lavender blooms in the area around Amman, Jordan, from March through May and can be found in local flower shops.

❧ *L. multifida*, with its feathery foliage, originates in North Africa and is known as Egyptian lavender.

❧ Lavender is widely cultivated for its aromatic flowers in England, France, Spain, Italy and other European countries. The essential oil of English lavender *(L. angustifolia* or *L. vera)* is widely used in aromatherapy.

❧ In Turkey and Egypt, lavender flowers are used for perfuming the bath.

❧ Lavender flowers are used to scent pillows and sachets.

❧ Lavender was one of the herbs brought to the New World by the Pilgrims.

LEMON BALM

Melissa officinalis
Lamiaceae (Mint) Family
Arabic: *al-melissa*
Other English: Balm, Melissa

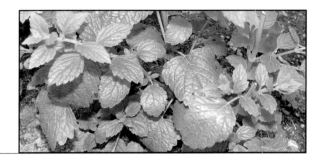

Lemon balm, or melissa, originated in the Middle East and has been cultivated in the region for more than 2,000 years. Arab medicine has long recommended melissa for its calming properties. The 11th-century medical genius Ibn Sina – known to his admiring European contemporaries as Avicenna – prescribed lemon balm for melancholy and even for heart problems.

The crushed leaves of melissa smell like lemons and contain most of the medicinal value of the plant (volatile oils, tannins and bitters). Not only is this plant a gentle and effective nerve tonic, but it also tastes delicious.

HOW TO USE

1. Chop the fresh leaves into salads.

2. Infuse the leaves to make a tea.

IN THE KITCHEN

To make melissa tea, pour boiling water over the leaves and cover tightly with a lid. Steep for 20 minutes. Strain and drink.

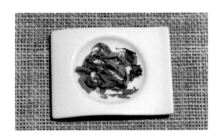

DID YOU KNOW?

🦎 Arab traders introduced lemon balm to Europe through Spain.

🦎 Today, Hungary, Egypt and Italy are major producers of the herb, and the United States is a leading producer of organically grown melissa and melissa essential oil.

🦎 In Germany, the famed alchemist Paracelsus called this herb the 'elixir of life,' and used it in a compound called *Primum Ens Melissae,* reputed to restore vigour and prolong life.

🦎 Lemon balm is reported to increase energy in the system by helping to release energy blocks and stress. It is relaxing, yet stimulating. It acts as an anti-depressant.

🦎 Melissa blended with chamomile and oats makes a delicious nervine tonic.

🦎 In Europe, lemon balm has been used as a salve for herpes simplex symptoms.

🦎 *Mother Earth News* recommends lemon balm as a homemade mosquito repellent, because its oil contains citronellal and other substances: 'just crush a handful of the delicious-smelling leaves in your hand and rub them on exposed skin.'

FAMILY REMEDIES ACROSS ARABIA

Melissa is excellent for stomach distress and general exhaustion because its effects are sedative, relaxing and mildly anti-spasmodic.

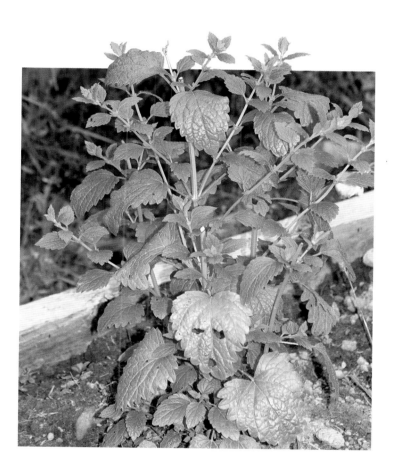

RESEARCH

A new study in the United Kingdom shows that *Melissa officinalis*, administered in capsules of dried leaf, can improve cognitive performance and mood and may therefore be a 'valuable adjunct' in the treatment of Alzheimer's disease. (Kennedy, D.O., et al. 'Modulation of mood and cognitive performance following acute administration of single doses of *Melissa officinalis* (Lemon balm) with human CNS nicotinic and muscarinic receptor-binding properties.' *Neuropsychopharmacology.* 2003 Oct; 28(10): 1871-81.)

Studies have shown that lemon balm prevents certain viruses from attaching to cells. Topical applications of lemon balm extracts have resulted in significant reduction of the severity and duration of herpes symptoms, oral and genital. (Wolbling, R.H., and K. Leonhardt. 'Local therapy of herpes simplex with dried extract from *Melissa officinalis.' Phytomedicine.* 1994; 1:25–31; Dimitrova, Z., et al. 'Antiherpes effect of Melissa officinalis L. extracts.' *Acta Microbiol. Bulg.* 1993; 29:65–72.)

LIME, DRIED

Citrus aurantifolia
Rutaceae (Citrus) Family
Arabic: *loomi, lumi, limun aswad*
Other English: Black Lime, Black Lemon

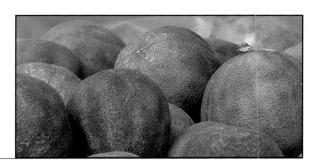

A newcomer to the Middle East, Karen felt confused as she approached the outdoor market. She had read in a Saudi cookbook that *loomi* was a term for 'dried, whole limes'. Yet she understood the Arabic term to be *limun aswad*, or black lemon. So, what was *loomi*? Lime or lemon? As she studied the baskets full of this dried fruit, she noted that it seemed closer in size to limes. She also observed that some *loomi* piles were a natural tan colour while others were blackened. It was time to get some answers.

Speaking to several shopkeepers, Karen learned that *loomi* – imported from Iran, India, Oman and Sudan – definitely meant dried lime. Ripe limes are boiled in salt-water and then dried until the interior turns dark (hence the name 'black lime' or 'black lemon'). Although light brown or tan in colour when dried naturally, *loomi* is often blackened because consumers in the Middle East have grown accustomed to this appearance. *Loomi* adds citrus fragrance and a sour tang to meats, legumes and other foods.

Pleased with her new knowledge, Karen purchased her first selection of *loomi* and hurried home to try some Arabian cooking.

HOW TO USE

1. Dry your own limes by rapidly boiling them for three minutes. Drain, then dry in the sun until completely dehydrated.

2. Puncture one end of a dried lime and include it in rice and meat dishes as a flavouring.

3. Grate or grind dried *loomi* into a powder and use it as a spice.

IN THE KITCHEN

The renowned *kabsa* dish calls for dried whole *loomi*, as do many rice and meat dishes. Saute powdered black lime with onion and put on top of *qursan* and *jarish* as a garnish.

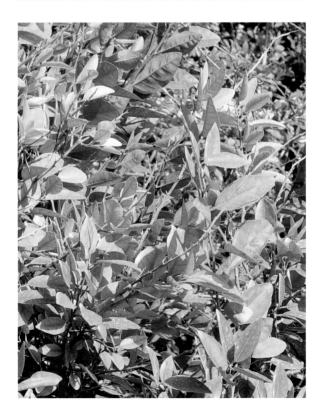

RECIPES	
	Chicken Kabsa, p. 190
	Matazeez, p. 192
	Jarish, p. 194
	Qursan, p. 194
	Mufallaq with Meat, p. 196
	Hasawi Rice with Shrimp, p. 197

FAMILY REMEDIES ACROSS ARABIA

Loomi is used to treat diarrhoea, colic and menstrual pain.

Colds and Coughs: Use lime with tea and honey. (Western KSA)

Colic: Soak *loomi* in water then bring to a boil. Strain and drink to reduce colic. (Eastern KSA)

Diarrhoea: Eat dry tea leaves. Also use *loomi* (black lime) and salt. (Eastern KSA) ✿ I use *loomi* to treat diarrhoea. Grill two *loomi*s. Then boil them in water. Strain and drink the liquid. (Eastern KSA) ✿ Use powdered *loomi* to treat diarrhoea. Remove seeds before grinding (seeds are bitter). (Eastern KSA)

Menstrual Pain: Soak *loomi* in water, then bring to a boil. Strain and drink to reduce menstrual pain. (Eastern KSA) ✿ Use cinnamon and *loomi*. (Eastern KSA)

DID YOU KNOW?

✿ In the Western Province of Saudi Arabia, *loomi* is called 'Bin Zuhair'.

✿ Bedouin women traditionally dyed their yarns with natural substances, including dried lime (*loomi*), henna, madder and pomegranate skins. Alum is used as the mordant and is available in bulk in local markets.

✿ In Northern India and Iran, powdered *loomi* is used to flavour rice, as a substitute for sumac. It is particularly popular with Indian basmati rice.

✿ Lime juice is sweeter than lemon juice.

✿ Limes are so fragrant that the oil from the skin is used in perfumery.

✿ Limes are rich in vitamin C. In the 17th century, limes were issued to British sailors to prevent the nutritional deficiency known as scurvy. As a result, British sailors, and later British emigrants to the US and Australia, became known as 'limeys'.

RESEARCH

Concentrated lime juice has been shown to have a modifying or regulating effect on certain immune functions. (Gharagozloo, M., and A. Ghaderi. 'Immunomodulatory effect of concentrated lime juice extract on activated human mononuclear cells.' *J Ethnopharmacol.* 2001 Sep; 77(1): 85-90.)

Iranian researchers report that concentrated lime juice extract has a significant effect countering the growth of certain human cancer cells. (Gharagozloo, M., et al. 'Effects of *Citrus aurantifolia* concentrated extract on the spontaneous proliferation of MDA-MB-453 and RPMI-8866 tumor cell lines.' *Phytomedicine.* 2002 Jul; 9(5): 475-7.)

MAHALEB CHERRY

Prunus mahaleb or *Cerasus mahaleb*
Rosaceae (Rose) Family
Arabic: *mahaleb, mahlab*
Other English: Rock Cherry, English
Cherry, St Lucie Cherry, Perfumed Cherry

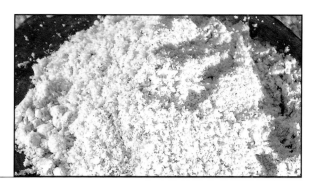

The most popular offering of the *Prunus mahaleb* – a deciduous tree that grows to a height of about 10 metres, or 35 feet – is the aromatic kernel obtained from its black cherry stones. When these kernels are dried and ground into a powder, they are used to flavour pastries throughout the Middle East and Turkey. Mahaleb is found in traditional Arabian markets either as dried fruits or as kernels.

HOW TO USE

Grind the dried kernel of the cherry stones into a fine powder.

IN THE KITCHEN

To ensure a fresh flavour, buy dried mahaleb kernels whole and then grind them into powder as needed. The kernels have a high lipid content and their powder can turn rancid rather quickly in storage.

BEAUTY TIP | Mahaleb Perfume, p 173.

DID YOU KNOW?

↬ In ancient times, mahaleb was one of the spices brought by Arab caravans to Constantinople and Alexandria, and from there to the cities of Greece. Today this distinctive, fruity spice, called *mahlepi* in Greek, is a traditional ingredient of *tsoureki* (braided Easter sweet bread), as well as holiday cakes and cookies.

↬ The physician Ibn Ridwan of 11th-century Egypt recommends oil of mahaleb as a 'warming aromatic'. When heated, the oil improves the quality of the air in a home on a cold day.

↬ Physician Ibn Sina (called Avicenna in the West), also writing in the 11th century, cites mahaleb as a 'simple drug which warms and does not purge'.

↬ Today, the perfumed cherry tree grows widely in Western Asia. It is found in some parts of Eastern and Central Europe.

↬ Mahaleb seeds were once regarded by the Turks as a traditional remedy for malaria.

↬ Mahaleb grows in many parts of the United States, where, because of its robust nature and resistance to disease, it is used as a cherry tree grafting stock.

↬ Mahaleb's use in foods and medicines is mostly limited to Greece, Turkey, Armenia and the Middle East.

FAMILY REMEDIES ACROSS ARABIA

Both the dried fruits and the kernels are sold for medicinal use. Arabian physicians have long used the small (1cm diameter) fruit of *Prunus mahaleb* to break up kidney stones and gallstones, promote drainage of urine, treat colic and iliac pains, and serve as an anti-nauseant, and used the dried kernels of the black cherry stones as a stomachic and for general weakness. Mahaleb powder has been used in skin and hair care applications.

Fever: To reduce temperatures of children, mix mahaleb powder with water and apply to the forehead. Within 20 minutes, the temperature should be lowered. (Central and Southern KSA)

Skin Cleanser: Use honey, lemon and mahaleb to clean the body naturally. (Northern KSA)

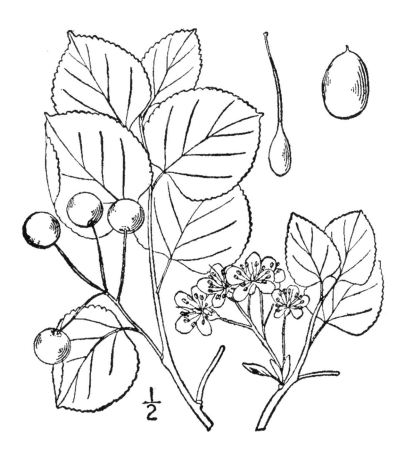

Prunus mahaleb L.

RESEARCH

Mahaleb contains an organic compound called coumarin, which has blood-thinning, anti-fungal and anti-tumour properties. Coumarin is used to make an oral anticoagulant medication. (El-Dakhakhny, M. 'Some coumarin constitutents of *Prunus mahaleb L.* fruit kernels. V.' *J Pharm Sci.* 1970 Apr; 59(4): 551-3.)

MANGROVE

Avicennia marina (A.officinalis)

Avicenniaceae or Verbenaceae (Verbena)
   Family

Arabic: *qurm, qirm, gurm, girm, shura*

Other English: Gray Mangrove, Black
   Mangrove

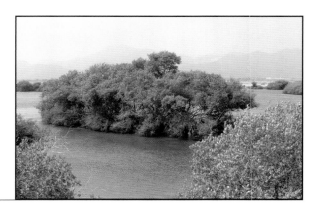

In May 2005, some 500 Saudi schoolchildren gathered on the beaches along Tarut Bay near Ras Tanura. They weren't there to swim. These boys and girls had come to plant thousands of mangrove tree seedlings in the sand not far from the waters of the Arabian Gulf. For many of the students, this was their first hands-on experience at protecting the local environment.

The mangrove seedling project, organized by Saudi Aramco with the help of local charities and the Ministry of Agriculture, is part of a wider environmental initiative to restore and maintain traditional habitats in the Gulf region.

Mangroves are salt-tolerant maritime trees that flourish in certain tropical and subtropical coastal areas, including those of Saudi Arabia and other Gulf countries. Mangroves grow in the sheltered intertidal zone between the land and the sea, in estuaries and sometimes on the tops of coral reefs.

Mangroves with their elaborate root systems help protect shorelines, sea grass beds and coral reefs; and prove a nursery for fish, shrimp and crabs; as well as food and sanctuary for littoral wildlife. Mangrove trees have respiratory roots called pneumatophores that rise up vertically from the mud and sand around the tree. These roots absorb atmospheric oxygen during low tides. Mangrove leaves range from light to dark green in colour and possess glands that excrete excess salt.

Mangrove trees are also found along the coast of Qatar, and at various lagoons and near-shore islands on the coast of the United Arab Emirates including Abu Dhabi, Umm

HOW TO USE

Along the Gulf coast of Saudi Arabia, Qatar and the UAE, mangrove trees have traditionally been a source of firewood, housing material, charcoal and fodder for camels and other animals. The wood burns very well, and makes good lumber. Medicinally, its unripe seeds and its leaves have been used in poultices for various skin disorders and diseases.

IN THE KITCHEN

Mangrove wood is seldom needed in the kitchen today because modernization has provided other sources of fuel. The edible parts of the plant do not figure in Gulf cuisine.

Khor Kalba, Sharjah, United Arab Emirates (above and below).

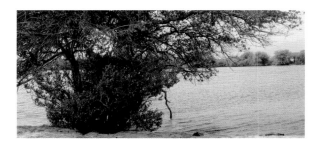

al-Qaiwain, Ras al-Khaima and Khor Kalba.

Khor Kalba, on the UAE's east coast and straddling the border with Oman, is reputed to be the oldest mangrove forest in Arabia. The large swamp is also a conservation reserve with abundant birdlife. Bird enthusiasts flock to this area because it is the only home of the rare white-collared kingfisher *(Halcyon chloris kalbaensis)*, which feeds mostly on the small crabs that thrive among the mangrove roots.

FAMILY REMEDIES ACROSS ARABIA

Abdominal Pain: Peppermint and sage are for abdominal pain. (Southern KSA) ✿ Use peppermint leaves for stomachache. It makes you feel fresh and makes your blood flow. (Northern KSA) ✿ Peppermint is for treating illnesses of the stomach and pain, as well as monthly period pains and gases. It calms a person down. (Eastern KSA) ✿ Peppermint. Boil it with tea or alone. It's used to relieve swelling in the abdomen. (Southern KSA) ✿ For a stomachache, use cumin and peppermint. Boil them in water and drink. (Northern KSA)

Childbirth: To strengthen a mother after childbirth, use fenugreek, cress, cinnamon, sage and peppermint. (KSA)

Colds or Coughs: Dried peppermint has been used for colds. (Eastern KSA) ✿ For colds or coughs, use peppermint or ginger in milk. (Northern KSA) ✿ We use ginger, mint, lemon, honey and black seed for coughs and colds. (Eastern KSA) ✿ Drink boiled basil with peppermint sweetened with lemon juice and crystalline sugar. (Eastern KSA) ✿ Use peppermint for swelling. (Northern KSA)

Colic: Boil equal quantities of anise, cumin and peppermint and add some crystalline sugar or honey. Then put 7 drops of black seed oil and drink while hot. It is good for colic. (Eastern KSA) ✿ Drink 1 spoonful of onion juice and one of vinegar to treat colic and put a mixture of shredded onion with peppermint oil or clove on the painful area. (Eastern KSA)

Flatulence (Intestinal Gas): Peppermint leaves are used as tea to remove gases. (Eastern KSA)

Headaches: Use peppermint, saffron, ginger and water (drink). (Southern KSA) ✿ Smell fresh mint. (Western KSA)

Indigestion: Take boiled peppermint sweetened with sugar. (Southern KSA) ✿ Boil mint sprigs and drink the liquid. (Western KSA) ✿ Boiled peppermint, wild thyme. (Central KSA) ✿ We use soaked peppermint and soaked basil. Also, boil an onion with its skin, then remove the skin and mash it in honey and eat in a sandwich. Also, for digestion, eat onion with date, fennel, black seed, thyme and cheese. (Eastern KSA) ✿ Use myrrh, *luqah* (from the date palm tree) and peppermint. (Eastern KSA)

Insomnia: Peppermint and basil. (Southern KSA) ✿ Boiled peppermint with milk. (Central KSA) ✿ Drink anise and peppermint. (Central KSA) ✿ Lemon juice or peppermint. Boil water with peppermint like tea. (Central KSA)

Menstrual Pain: Drink hot peppermint and cinnamon – and coffee bean peelings. (Southern KSA) ✿ Cinnamon helps to stimulate the menses if it's late. (Southern KSA)

Sore Throats: Use 1 tablespoon of honey in $^1/_2$ cup water and mix, then gargle three times a day. Also, drink soaked peppermint. Also, put a hot onion compress around the neck and above the larynx. Gargle onion juice with honey three times a day. (Eastern KSA)

DID YOU KNOW?

ى More than 600 different types of mint have been classified around the world, most of them variants or hybrids of some 25 well-defined species. There are two primary cultivated mints: peppermint *(Mentha piperita)* and spearmint *(Mentha spicata)*.

ى Peppermint *(M. piperita)* is an English hybrid from water mint *(M. aquatica)* and spearmint *(M. spicata)*, and is well-established in Egypt and throughout North Africa. As a rule, peppermint can be substituted in recipes for any other type of aromatic mint, but the reverse is not always true.

ى Mint has been used in many cultures as a digestive and to disguise the unpleasant taste of other medicines.

ى In ancient Babylon, mint was prescribed for a variety of ailments, including halitosis, coughs, heartburn, excessive salivation, swellings, and eye and ear problems.

ى Al-Kindi, the 9th-century Arab physician, used mint in an oxymel (a honey-vinegar syrup) for quartan malarial fever, and recommended it for stomach and liver pain.

ى In medieval Syriac medicine, 'river mint' (probably *Mentha aquatica*) was used to bring on menstrual flow.

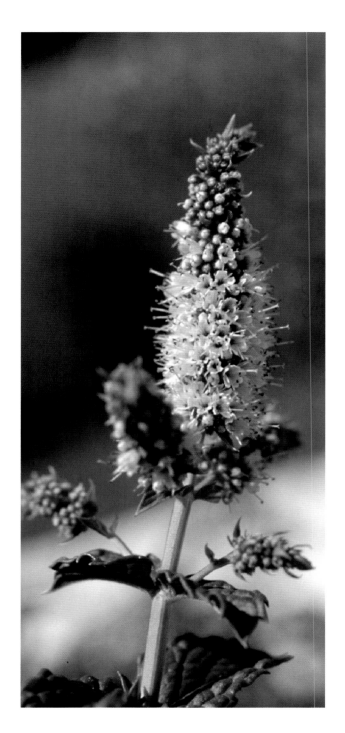

ى Al-Baghdadi, in his 13th-century *Kitab al-Tabikh* (A Baghdad Cookery Book), recommends certain sauces to 'cleanse the palate of greasiness, to appetize, to assist the digestion, and to stimulate the banqueter'. One of these sauces is *Na'na' Mukhallal* (Mint in Vinegar), in which 'the mint has absorbed the sourness of the vinegar so that the latter has lost its sharpness'.

RESEARCH

Peppermint oil has been shown to inhibit and kill herpes simplex virus types 1 and 2, and may be suitable for topical therapeutic use as a virucidal agent in recurrent herpes infections. (Schuhmacher, A., et al. 'Virucidal effect of peppermint oil on the enveloped viruses herpes simplex virus type 1 and type 2 in vitro.' *Phytomedicine.* 2003; 10(6-7): 504-10.)

Mentha piperita has been shown to protect the intestines of laboratory mice from radiation damage. (Samarth, R.M., et al. '*Mentha piperita* (Linn) leaf extract provides protection against radiation induced alterations in intestinal mucosa of Swiss albino mice.' *Indian J Exp Biol.* 2002 Nov; 40(11): 1245-9.)

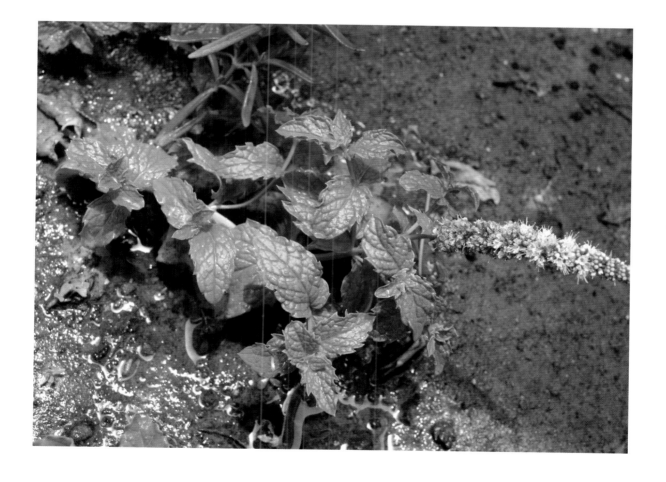

MYRRH

Commiphora myrrha or *C. molmol* or
   Balsamodendron myrrha
Burseraceae (Frankincense and Myrrh)
   Family
Arabic: *murr, murrah*

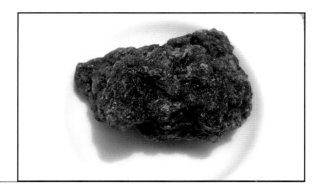

Myrrh is collected from the stems of bushy shrubs found growing in southern Arabia and Somalia. A granular secretion exits the stem through natural fissures, or cuts, as a pale yellow liquid. It then hardens to a reddish-brown mass. It can be found in different sizes in the marketplace, most pieces being the size of large marbles or walnuts.

While shopping in a traditional market, one simply needs to ask for '*murr.*' The word myrrh means 'bitter' in Arabic. A kilogram of myrrh may be purchased for about 90 riyals ($24) in the local markets of Arabia.

Myrrh is an antiseptic, an astringent and a stimulant, and has other medicinal properties. As one of the best antiseptics known, it is commonly applied to disinfect wounds. In fact, celebrated herbalist Jethro

---

HOW TO USE

1. Soak myrrh granules in water for 2-3 days and then drink the strained liquid.

2. Swallow small granules like pills.

3. Burn as incense.

IN THE KITCHEN

Many families keep a glass jar of myrrh covered with water in the refrigerator. Then, when this remedy is called for, the liquid is strained and ready to consume.

Kloss (1863-1946) left the legacy of Kloss liniment. He recommended putting 2 ounces of gum myrrh into a quart of rubbing alcohol along with 1 ounce of golden seal root and one half ounce of cayenne pepper and letting it stand for a week or 10 days, shaking it every day, and then straining prior to use. This liniment is healing for open wounds, cuts, scratches, bruises, sprains and any purpose for which liniment is required.

Part of a tableau in Queen Hatshepsut's funerary temple at Deir el-Bahri, which shows a myrrh tree from the land of Punt being borne back to Egypt.

FAMILY REMEDIES ACROSS ARABIA

Although it has an unpleasant bitter taste, myrrh is used to alleviate inflammation in the body. Myrrh water is an excellent mouthwash and is helpful for mouth sores or blisters, sore throats, bronchial congestion and other conditions requiring an antiseptic astringent.

Myrrh is used by women after the delivery of a baby. New mothers sit for about 15 minutes in a myrrh/salt water bath. Myrrh is also flammable and may be used as an incense.

Abdominal Pain: People drink myrrh water for abdominal pain. New mothers drink it after delivery. (Southern KSA) ✿ Put 3-4 pieces of myrrh in a ¹/₄ or ¹/₂ litre of hot water. Leave it for one night or more. Then, drink the water. It is a medicine for stomachache and skin infection and it acts like an antibiotic. (Central KSA) ✿ Myrrh is for stomachaches and is used by soaking it in room-temperature water. Leave it for three hours. Then drink its water. (Eastern KSA) ✿ Add powdered myrrh to water and drink it down quickly – it's very bitter! (Socotra, Yemen)

Burn: Soak myrrh in a small amount of water. It is put on burns to reduce scars and to help in quickly healing wounds and to remove warts. (Southern KSA)

Chest Complaint: Put myrrh in water. Leave for an hour until water is white. Drink without myrrh [strained] because it's good for your chest. It is an antibiotic. (KSA)

Childbirth: I used myrrh after giving a caesarean birth to my son. I put the myrrh next to the wound to help it heal. I also used myrrh orally for the first 40 days after my delivery. I would soak it in water overnight then drink about one small Arabic coffee cup of the liquid every morning, adding one teaspoon of honey to get rid of its very bitter taste. (Western KSA) ✿ Use fenugreek, cress, myrrh and *laban* to strengthen a mother after childbirth. (Eastern KSA)

Colic: Add a little powdered myrrh to milk and feed it to the baby to ease a distended abdomen. (Socotra, Yemen)

Colds and Coughs: Use myrrh and soup as well as hot water with salt. (Southern KSA)

Cuts: Myrrh is very good to have if you have external cuts. It makes them get better quickly. (Central KSA) ✿ Cover the cut with a little myrrh after soaking it in a little water for 3-4 hours. (Southern KSA)

Digestive System: We use myrrh for digestive system diseases. Also we use frankincense and myrrh for those with diabetes and hypertension because it reduces high sugar levels in the blood. (Eastern KSA)

Continued overleaf

FAMILY REMEDIES ACROSS ARABIA (*cont.*)

General Health: We use myrrh, frankincense for so many remedies – for example, to treat sores, appendicitis pain after an operation, boils, stomachaches and the colon. Soak myrrh stones in water. Then place the myrrh water on the painful area for boils or drink. (Central KSA) ✿ Myrrh and frankincense are put in water and drunk at bedtime. (Southern KSA) ✿ We take myrrh for colic, sadness, constipation, diarrhoea, nausea and inflammations. (Eastern KSA) ✿ Myrrh is for cleaning the stomach and removing blood clots from inside your body. (Northern KSA)

Infection: I use frankincense and myrrh continually for infections and as a preventative medicine for any kind of cancer. (Western KSA) ✿ Use myrrh as an antibiotic. Put 2-3 pieces in hot water. Allow to cool. Internal and external use. (Central KSA) ✿ I use myrrh as treatment for all diseases because it's considered as an antibiotic. (Eastern KSA) ✿ We use frankincense and myrrh and myrrh is more powerful and useful than antibiotics. It cures inflammations. It is said, 'A free woman (not a slave) doesn't stay up at night when she has myrrh at home.' Because with God's will it cures pains. (Central KSA)

Menstrual Pain: I use frankincense and myrrh whenever I have stomach or body aches or during my period. I soak them in water for a while, then use the water for treatment. (Eastern KSA) ✿ My grandmother used to have *bukhoor* (incense) of myrrh for dysmenorrhea. Apply it cool on the vagina. (Eastern KSA) ✿ Use myrrh as a medicine for female disorders. (Yemen)

Newborn Care: In the past, myrrh oil was wiped on a new baby's navel. Nowadays they use medical sterilizers. (Bahrain) ✿ Massage the newborn's navel with the pit of a date with myrrh and kohl. (Southern KSA)

Sore Throat: Myrrh is used to treat sore throats. Put myrrh in a cup of hot coffee and drink, or soak myrrh in a small amount of water. (Southern KSA) ✿ Gargle with hot water and salt or drink a little diluted soaked myrrh. (Southern KSA) ✿ I use myrrh to relieve a sore throat and kill germs. (Western KSA)

Wound: Myrrh is used to help heal wounds, minor burns, and incisions from simple surgical operations. (Southern KSA) ✿ There is a process called *shammam*: Hold pieces of myrrh, pre-soaked in water, about 3 inches from a cut for 3-4 minutes. Do this three times a day. It heals wounds from surgery. (Central KSA) ✿ Myrrh is used as an antibiotic. Add a small spoonful of myrrh to a cup of hot water and let sit for one night. The next morning, take one sip before breakfast and pour a few drops on the wound after surgery or wipe it with cotton to help the wound dry fast and protect it from germs. (Northern KSA) ✿ Myrrh quickly closes sores. Mix with henna for pain in the foot. (Eastern KSA)

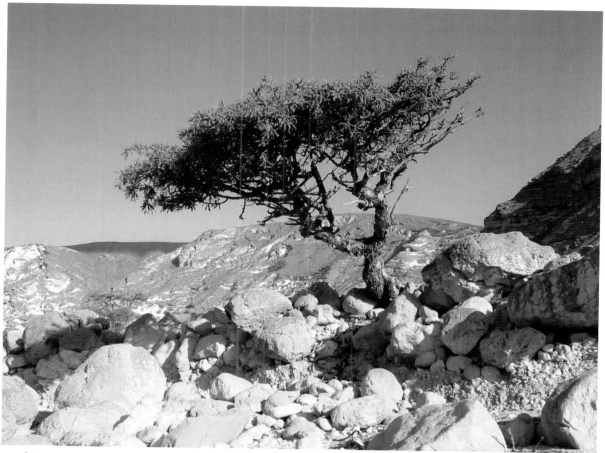

Frankincense tree, Oman.

RESEARCH

Scientific tests have shown myrrh to possess significant antibacterial and anti-inflammatory properties. (El Ashry, E.S., et al. 'Components, therapeutic value and uses of myrrh.' *Pharmazie*. 2003 Mar; 58(3): 163-8; Tipton, D.A., et al. 'In vitro cytotoxic and anti-inflammatory effects of myrrh oil on human gingival fibroblasts and epithelial cells.' *Toxicol In Vitro*. 2003 Jun; 17(3): 301-10.)

A medical survey in Saudi Arabia showed that almost 18 per cent of diabetic patients attending outpatient clinics in four major hospitals in Riyadh used herbs to treat their diabetes. The most common herbs were myrrh, black seed, *helteet* (asafoetida), fenugreek and aloes. Almost three-quarters of the herb users did not inform their doctors. (Al Rowais, N.A. 'Herbal medicine in the treatment of diabetes mellitus.' *Saudi Med J*. 2002 Nov; 23(11): 1327-31.)

NAKHWA

Trachyspermum ammi, Carum ajowan,
  Carum copticum, Ammi copticum
Apiaceae/Umbelliferae (Parsley) Family
Arabic: *nakhwa, nankha, nanakhwah*
Hindi: *ajwain, ajwan, ajowan*
Other English: Bishop's Weed

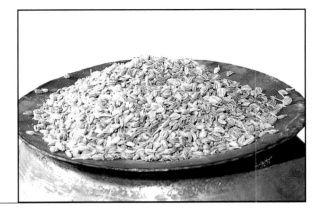

The *hawaaj* (herbalist) led Colin over to the spice counter and showed him the tiny, brownish-gray seeds. 'These seeds are similar in appearance to caraway and cumin,' he said, 'but they are slightly more curved in shape. We call them *nakhwa* or *ajwain*. They were used as medicine by the ancient Greeks and Arabs and are still considered a natural remedy for a variety of complaints. You can buy the aromatic seeds as well as a distillate obtained from the seeds. Both are excellent for treating stomach wind.'

HOW TO USE

1. Release the aroma of the seeds before use by rubbing between your fingertips, crushing with a mortar and pestle, or gently stirring while warming in a frying pan.

2. Use seeds whole or grind them into powder form.

IN THE KITCHEN

Nakhwa is sometimes added to traditional Arabic coffee. In addition to adding a unique flavour, it is believed to soften the impact of coffee on the stomach and reduce the effects of caffeine. In fact, some people across Arabia drink boiled *nakhwa* as a substitute for Arabic coffee to totally eliminate the negative effects of coffee.

RECIPE	*Arabic coffee with nakhwa, p. 179*

RESEARCH

Ethnobotanist James Duke mentions the use of *Trachyspermum ammi* for gastrosis (stomach complaints) and also reports that it enhances appetite and is also helpful for urinary problems.

Nakhwa (ajwain) oil has been shown to counteract certain harmful bacteria and to inhibit the growth of various microorganisms. (Saxena, A.P., and R.K. Singh. 70th Session of Ind. Sci. Congress, Abstr. 87, 1983.)

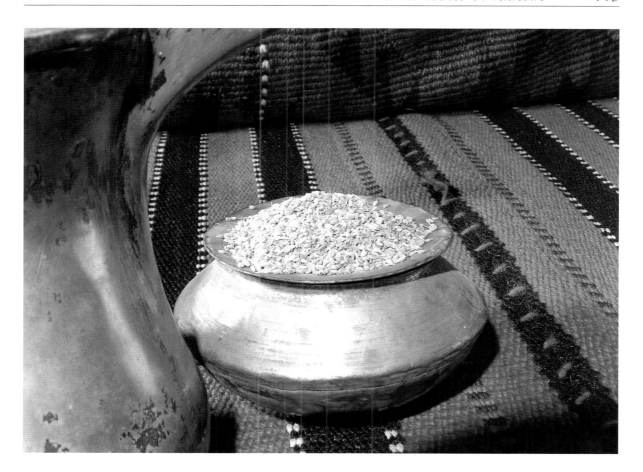

FAMILY REMEDIES ACROSS ARABIA

Breastfeeding: Mothers are advised to drink [boiled] *nakhwa* to increase milk flow. (Central KSA)

Stomach Pain: Add 1-2 teaspoons of *nakhwa* seeds to one cup boiling water. Steep for 5 minutes, strain and drink. (Western KSA)

DID YOU KNOW?

෴ Like black seed *(Nigella sativa)*, *nakhwa* is a popular ingredient in many herbal medicinal blends.

෴ The ancient Sumerians described *nakhwa* as a 'plant of the mountain'.

෴ *Nakhwa* is grown in Pakistan, Afghanistan, Iran, India and Egypt.

෴ Though more commonly cultivated today in Asia, *nakhwa* is actually of African origin, and some Arabs call it 'Ethiopian cumin' *(al-kammun al-habashi)*.

෴ Al-Kindi (c. 800-870 AD) used *nakhwa* in a preparation for haemorrhoids.

෴ *Nakhwa* seeds yield 40-55 per cent thymol, a valuable crystalline phenol extracted for medicinal purposes. In the West, thymol is used in some cough medicines.

NEEM

Azadirachta indica
Meliaceae (Mahogany) Family
Arabic: *neem*
Other English: Nim, Margosa Tree

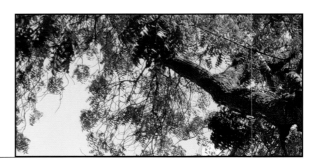

There are now thousands of trees growing throughout the Red Sea port city of Jeddah – in parks, along thoroughfares, in villa gardens and other irrigated areas. But up until 1948, there was only one tree in the entire city – the *neem* tree in front of the famous Bait Naseef or Naseef House *(pictured opposite)*. This house in Old Jeddah, with its classic *mashrabiyya* windows, is today a museum. And the original *neem* tree still stands in front of it. The tree became so famous that it was eventually incorporated into the museum's address: PO Box 3, the House with a Tree!

Today *neem* trees are found in most of Saudi Arabia's larger cities. They are used for landscaping purposes at many of the Kingdom's airports and government buildings. The *neem* tree is considered a natural air purifier, removing toxic gases and substances from the air and releasing life-giving oxygen.

Muslim pilgrims first brought neem to Arabia from the Indian subcontinent, where it has long been regarded as a 'wonder plant' with a wide range of medicinal uses. *Neem* is used to treat gum disease, skin conditions, ulcers, high blood pressure, diabetes, malaria and other ailments. *Neem* seeds and leaves are known to have antiviral, antifungal and antiseptic properties.

Traditional Indian medicinal uses of neem have become fairly widespread in Saudi Arabia and other Gulf countries, in part because of the presence of many South Asian expatriates. As a result, many *neem*-based products, including soap and toothpaste, are sold in the Gulf region.

HOW TO USE

1. Brew the dried leaves as tea.

2. Chew the fresh leaves for oral and digestive health.

3. Make a poultice from an infusion of the leaves.

IN THE KITCHEN

Put three or four dried neem leaves in an 8-oz. cup of hot water and let steep for a few minutes to make tea.

RESEARCH

Neem has been shown to possess anti-malarial activity. Leaf extracts are reportedly as effective as such conventional malaria treatments as quinine and chloroquine. Some studies show that even chloroquine-resistant strains of malaria are sensitive to *neem*. (MacKinnon, S., et al. 'Antimalarial activity of tropical Meliaceae extracts and gedunin derivatives.' *J Nat Prod.* 1997 Apr; 60(4): 336-41; Dhar, R., et al. 'Inhibition of the growth and development of asexual and sexual stages of drug-sensitive and resistant strains of the human malaria parasite *Plasmodium falciparum* by *Neem* (*Azadirachta indica*) fractions.' *J Ethnopharmacol.* 1998 May; 61(1): 31-9.)

New research shows that *neem* extract has a significant effect in controlling stomach ulcers in albino rats. (Raji, Y., et al. 'Effects of *Azadirachta indica* extract on gastric ulceration and acid secretion in rats.' *J Ethnopharmacol.* 2004 Jan; 90(1):167-70.)

FAMILY REMEDIES ACROSS ARABIA

In addition to *miswak* from the arak tree, natural toothbrushes from the tender twigs of the *neem* tree are valued for keeping the gums and teeth strong and healthy and preventing pyorrhea.

Skin Problems: Soak *neem* leaves in water and apply the water to rashes and other skin problems. (Eastern KSA)

DID YOU KNOW?

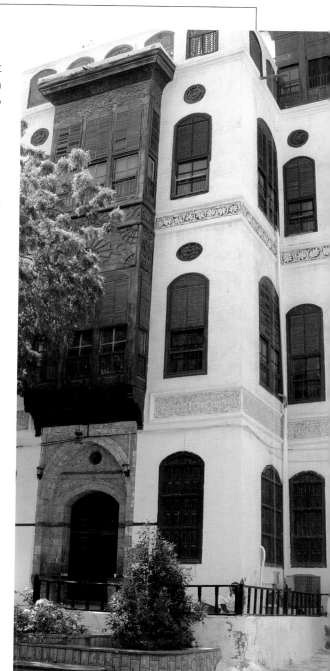

✑ The *neem* tree, native to India, was introduced in West Africa in the early 20th century in a bid to halt the expansion of the Sahara Desert. The tree has also been introduced to Saudi Arabia, South America, Central America, Australia, Mauritius and Fiji. It is now also grown in the United States, in such states as Florida, Arizona and California.

✑ In India, *neem* is sometimes called the 'village pharmacy' because of its multiplicity of medical uses. It has long been used in traditional Indian medicine and Ayurveda. In ancient Sanskrit, *neem* is known as *sarva roga nivarini,* 'the curer of all ailments.'

✑ *Neem* twigs are used by millions of Indians as an antiseptic toothbrush. Its oil is used in the preparation of toothpaste and soap.

✑ All parts of the *neem* tree – bark, roots, leaves, wood, flowers and fruits – have health benefits. The bark, including root bark, is a bitter tonic, stimulant and antiseptic. It stops secretions and bleeding, and controls spasms. The leaves, in a poultice, are a popular treatment for skin disorders, including psoriasis and eczema. The leaves are also powdered and consumed to treat stomach problems.

✑ While *neem* is safe for humans, animals and birds, it is lethal for many insects and is used as an insecticide. Dried leaves are sometimes kept in cupboards and cabinets to protect clothes, books, etc., from worms and insects. The pesticidal powers of *neem* seeds have been used by India's farmers for centuries.

✑ In Madagascar, *neem* leaves are chewed by women as a contraceptive. In other African countries, such as Ghana and Gambia, the liquid from boiled *neem* leaves is consumed during the first trimester of pregnancy to induce abortion.

NETTLE, DWARF

Urtica urens
Urticaceae (Nettle) Family
Arabic: *gurrais, qurrays, qurrais, qurras, hurqa, hariq, hurraiq*

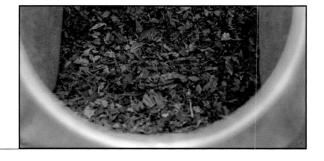

Dwarf nettle has been identified in the central and southern regions of Arabia. Dwarf nettle is a smaller relative of *Urtica dioica*, or stinging nettle, and possesses similar properties. The two species often grow together and in such cases are hard to distinguish from one another.

Dwarf nettles and others of their genus have various food and medicinal uses. Nettle contains a rich supply of such minerals as iron, silica, potassium, sulphur and manganese, as well as vitamins A and C. Nettle leaf tea is said to be a powerful tonic, packed with vitamins and minerals. The vitamin C content helps the body absorb the iron.

According to the 11th-century Spanish pharmacologist Ibn Biklarish, there are two kinds of nettle, *al-hurraiq* and *al-qurrais*. *Hurraiq* is 'coarser, blacker, with wider leaves'. *Qurrais* is known in Persian as '*artiqin*, which is also called the eye of the snake'.

HOW TO USE

1. Wash and boil the leaves. Cook and eat like spinach or use in soup.

2. Dry the leaves to make tea.

[NOTE: Always wear gloves when handling raw nettle. When touched, the bristly hairs of the plant inject an irritant substance under the skin. The sting disappears upon cooking.]

IN THE KITCHEN

In southern Saudi Arabia, henna *(Lawsonia inermis)* and nettle, washed and boiled, are added to wheat flour and eaten.

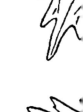

RESEARCH

Urtica urens leaf extracts are reportedly effective in treating rheumatoid arthritis. (Schulze-Tanzil, G. et al. 'Effects of the antirheumatic remedy hox alpha – a new stinging nettle leaf extract – on matrix metalloproteinases in human chondrocytes in vitro.' *Histol Histopathol*. 2002 Apr; 17(2): 477-85.)

Dwarf nettle tincture is one of the active ingredients in an effective homeopathic gel to treat mosquito bites. (Hill, N., et al. 'The efficacy of Prikweg gel in the treatment of insect bites: a double-blind, placebo-controlled clinical trial.' *Pharm World Sci*. 1996 Jan; 18(1): 35-41.)

FAMILY REMEDIES ACROSS ARABIA

Dwarf nettle has been used in medicine as an irritant. A decoction of the root applied to the scalp is considered a treatment for baldness. A decoction of the plant is used to treat diarrhoea. Dwarf nettle is also used to treat rheumatic problems and colds.

Hair Care: To strengthen and stimulate the growth of hair and make it shiny and silky, boil chamomile with water and add nettle. Leave it boiling then mix it with henna (powdered). Then leave it until it becomes warm then put on hair and leave for 4-6 hours. Then, wash the hair very well and apply some olive oil and rub hair and scalp. Then, wash with shampoo. (Eastern KSA)

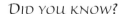

DID YOU KNOW?

☙ In Arabic, *qurras* means 'stinger' and *qurrais* means 'little stinger.' *Hariq* means 'fire,' *hurqa* means 'burning' and *hurraiq* means 'little burner.'

☙ Nettles of various species have provided fibres for cloth and paper since the Bronze Age.

☙ In Arabia, the name *qurrays* is sometimes applied to two other, unrelated plant species: *Aaronsohnia factorovskyi* and *Trigonella hamosa*. Botanist James. P. Mandaville says desert Bedouins eat *A. factorovskyi* raw and also use it in dried sour milk cakes. In 1928, explorer Alois Musil reported that in Northern Arabia, *qurrays* was *T. hamosa,* which he said Bedouins often consumed uncooked as a salad herb.

☙ Avicenna (980-1037 AD) prescribed nettle seeds to treat kidney stones and gallstones. Both Avicenna and Ibn Biklarish agreed that nettle is a powerful aphrodisiac if eaten with onions and egg yolks.

☙ Ibn Biklarish mentions many medicinal uses of dwarf nettle (*qurrais*) in the Middle Ages. The leaves were pounded, mixed with salt and used as a poultice for cancerous ulcers, 'filthy' ulcers, nerve pain, abscesses and eye swellings. The mixture, applied to the nostrils, was also said to stop nosebleeds.

☙ Dwarf nettle allays urethral and cystic irritation and has also been found efficient in uterine haemorrhage. It is also known as a galactagogue.

PETROLEUM

Arabic: *naft, batrul*

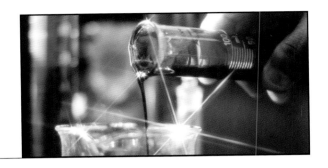

Although few people are aware of it today, petroleum was once considered an effective natural remedy not only in the Middle East but in many parts of the world.

While the modern petroleum industry is approximately a century and a half old, the practice of collecting and using petroleum dates back thousands of years

Oil upwellings and gas vents were known anciently in present-day Kuwait, Iraq, Iran, Azerbaijan, Turkmenistan and Uzbekistan. Natural deposits of thickened petroleum (also called bitumen) seeped from openings on land, or floated to the surface of lakes. It was easy to gather and was used as a building material, waterproofing material, lubricant, adhesive, art object, medicine, fuel, illuminant, fumigant and even as a weapon.

(Much of the historical information on petroleum in these pages was gleaned from the Saudi Aramco Exhibit in Dhahran, and from a series of articles on "Ancient Oil Industries" by Zayn Bilkadi, in Aramco World *magazine, 1994-95.)*

HOW TO USE

The All-Encompassing Dictionary (Al-Qamus al-Muhit), written in Mecca in the 15th century by Abu Tahir al-Fayruzabadi, a scholar of Persian descent, contains a remarkable section on the uses of oil. It reveals that oil was commonly sold as medicine, as a fuel for lighting, and that it was used as an incendiary in a type of military flame thrower.

IN THE KITCHEN

Early travellers to the Middle East reported two ways in which local inhabitants used seeping petroleum as fuel. One method combined bitumen with ashes. The compound was then burned to cook food. In the second method, tubes were inserted in the ground near a gas seep and ignited at the tops. Three or four such flames boiled water or roasted food.

Nowadays, petrolatum (petroleum jelly) – a neutral, odourless, tasteless unguent distilled from petroleum and then purified – is sometimes used in bakery products as a release agent. Petrolatum meets US Food and Drug Administration (FDA) requirements for medicinal, cosmetic-formula and animal-feed use, and is also approved for direct contact with food.

RESEARCH

Medicinal vaseline (petrolatum) can protect exposed skin in industrial situations for up to six hours, according to a Russian study. (Shulakov, N.A., et al. '[Vaseline protection of the skin from the effects of the sealant Uniherm-6.]' *Gig Tr Prof Zabol.* 1990; (12): 43-4.)

FAMILY REMEDIES ACROSS ARABIA

Written descriptions of petroleum's alleged healing powers date from 2,000 years ago, although its traditional medicinal use is probably much older. Oil-and-water-baths were supposed to strengthen the body. Ointments of bitumen and other chemicals were often applied to sores or broken bones. Other petroleum preparations acted as antidotes to poison, fumigants, disinfectants or laxatives. Petroleum was even prescribed as an insecticide and remedy for cattle plague.

The Book of the Powers of Remedies, a medical text prepared by Masarjawah, a prominent physician living in Basra, Iraq, during the 7th century AD, described the benefits of ingesting oil for fighting disease and infection. Masarjawah wrote: 'Warm naphtha, especially water-white naphtha, when ingested in small doses, is excellent for suppressing cough, for asthma, bladder discomfort and arthritis.'

The All-Encompassing Dictionary states: 'The best grade of naphtha is the water-white. It is a good solvent, a diluent and an expectorant. Taken internally, it relieves cramps and aches of the belly, and, when applied topically, it can soothe skin rashes and infections.'

Vicks VapoRub, a nasal decongestant, cough suppressant and topical analgesic, contains petrolatum. The special consistency of petrolatum acts as a vehicle for the active ingredients and also helps to prevent moisture loss from the skin.

Other salves, suppositories and cosmetic products also benefit from the consistency contributed by petrolatums.

Coughs or Colds: We rub the chest with olive oil and a little Vicks. (Central KSA)

Cuts: Garlic for ant bites and Vicks for cuts. White ashes for cuts. (Northern KSA)

Headaches: Rub Vicks on the upper part of your face. (Central KSA)

Sore Throats: Honey or Vicks [for external treatment]. (Southern KSA) ❧ You put Vicks on your neck. (Central KSA). ❧ Rub [throat] with Vicks, then take a piece of cloth and wrap it around your neck. Then pull the cloth up, rubbing it upwards on the neck as much you can stand it, 5-6 times. It's painful. (Central KSA)

Stomachache: Cauterize feet with a hot knife. Then rub with Vicks and warm your feet by wearing socks, and you can drink something called *ishriq* (senna). (Central KSA)

DID YOU KNOW?

⤳ First recorded use of petroleum as an illuminant dates back to the beginning of the first century AD. People in Arab cultures used petroleum for lamp fuel in homes, markets and mosques as early as the ninth century AD. Kerosene lamps were in existence in the Muslim world more than a thousand years before they became known in the West.

⤳ For thousands of years, throughout the Middle East, asphalt (or 'bitumen') from natural deposits was mixed with clay or grass to provide the mortar to bind brick walls. Natural asphalt also went into the construction and finishing of homes and palaces, dikes, piers and roads.

⤳ Ancient mariners waterproofed their boats by smearing the woven and bundled reeds (and later wood) with bitumen.

⤳ Akkadian clay tablets from about 2200 BC referred to crude oil as *naptu*, from which derives the root of the later Arabic word for the substance, *naft*.

⤳ The Middle Eastern custom of ingesting crude oil and bitumen for medicinal purposes began in ancient Mesopotamia, spread to Egypt, and was continued by the Romans.

⤳ Ancient Egyptians used a bitumen mixture called *mumiya* ('mummy') to embalm their dead. In the 12th century, medieval Europeans learned that an oil could be extracted from this substance that Ibn al-Baytar and other Muslim physicians claimed was of great medicinal value. In time the oil was forgotten, but 'mummy' powder became an apothecary staple. Fake 'mummy' was produced domestically in Europe and traded until the 18th century.

⤳ Avicenna (11th century) recommended bitumen, a tar-like substance from the Dead Sea or the Black Sea, for various external medicinal uses. He identifies bitumen as one of the 'simple drugs which warm and do not purge'.

⤳ In 18th-century Baku and other parts of the Caspian Sea region, herbalists used petroleum to treat rheumatism, skin diseases and kidney stones. Veterinarians employed it as a dip to combat parasites and treat skin diseases in cattle and other farm animals.

⤳ Petroleum is used today in homeopathic medicine to treat motion sickness, eczema and other skin problems, nausea and diarrhoea.

⤳ Shilajit is the name of a traditional bitumen medicine from India. It has been used as a kidney tonic as well as an aid to increase sexual energy. Shilajit is believed to transport nutrients deep into tissue and to remove toxins. It is a treatment to improve memory and the ability to handle stress, reduce recovery time in muscle, bone and nerve injuries, stimulate the immune system and reduce chronic fatigue.

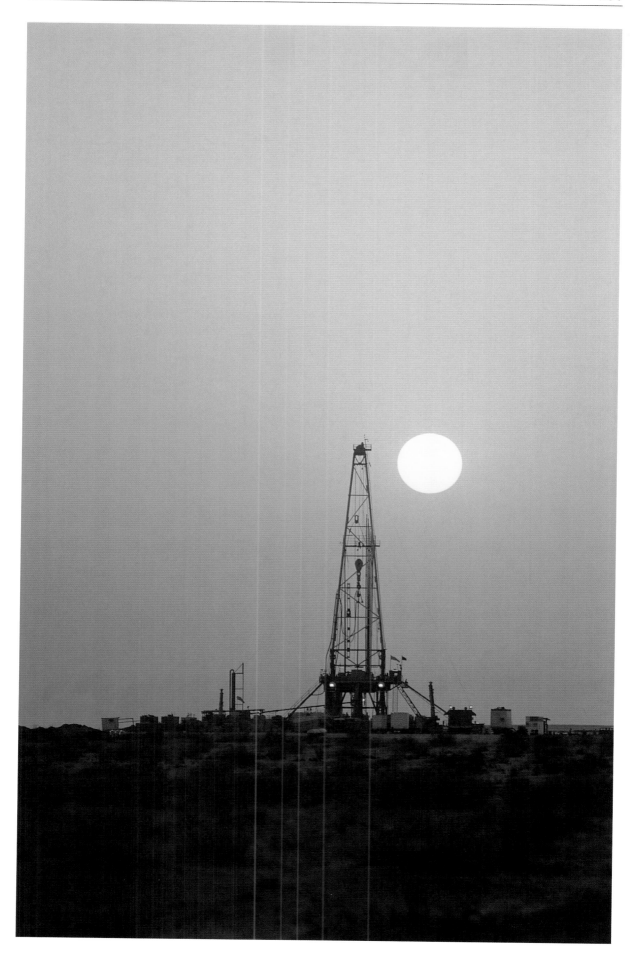

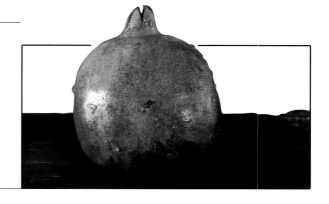

POMEGRANATE

Punica granatum
Lythraceae/Punicaceae Family
Arabic: *rumman*

When British explorer H. St John Philby visited an oasis in the southern Najd region of Arabia in the early 20th century, he observed widespread cultivation of date and tamarisk trees, cotton bushes, onions, beans, okra, figs, apricots, grapes, melons, lemons, garlic and ... pomegranates.

While native to Iran and its neighboring countries, the pomegranate was cultivated in ancient times all around the Mediterranean and throughout the Arabian Peninsula. It is a deciduous tree or large shrub that produces excellent fruit under semiarid conditions. Nowadays, Taif, Saudi Arabia's 'Summer Capital,' has a reputation for producing pomegranates of the highest quality.

| RECIPE | Arugula and Pomegranate Salad, p. 185 |

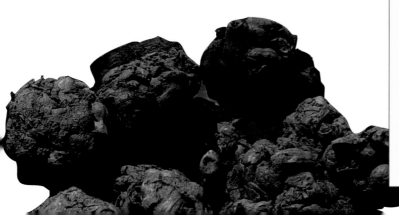

Pomegranate balls for sale in Qatif, Saudi Arabia.

HOW TO USE

1. Eat the fleshy seeds to enjoy a delicious, slightly tart flavour.

2. Dry the seeds and use in cooking.

3. Extract the juice from the seeds for a refreshing drink or as a flavouring agent in cooking.

4. Dry the outer peelings and crush them for culinary, cosmetic or medicinal purposes.

5. Boil pomegranate peelings in water, then strain and drink the liquid; if more concentrated, the liquid can be used as a dye for clothes.

6. Dry the peelings, then grind and mix with henna to make it darker and provide skin nourishment.

IN THE KITCHEN

Pomegranate seeds have a sweet-sour taste. Crushed or whole, they often garnish salads, couscous, hummus and other Mid-Eastern dishes. Dried pomegranate seeds and pomegranate syrup are also popular in cooking. Pomegranate juice is a refreshing drink on hot summer days. Pomegranate juice stains indelibly, so it is wise to wear protective clothing when cooking with it.

Pomegranate peelings that have been dried and crushed are sometimes mixed with water to form a ball. These dark-coloured pomegranate balls are available in local traditional markets. Add small amounts (not the entire ball!) to liquid when cooking fish. It flavours the dish and is believed to promote lactation for nursing mothers.

If stored in a cool, dry place, pomegranates will keep for months after harvesting. Although the rind shrinks and loses its lustrous colour, the flavour improves over time and the seeds become more edible and tender.

FAMILY REMEDIES ACROSS ARABIA

Powdered pomegranate peelings are used on burns and to treat infection on external cuts and wounds. Soaked pomegranate peelings are used for sore throats, stomachaches, and indigestion. To treat indigestion, pomegranate peelings are dried, then boiled, and the water drunk. Rose water can be added for flavour. Pomegranates soaked in boiled water are used with honey for heart trouble.

Pomegranate fruit rind and bark contain pelletierene alkaloids, elligatannins and triterpenoids. The alkaloids are highly toxic, so internal use of the rind or bark should take place only under professional supervision.

Burns: Apply powdered pomegranate peelings; soaked myrrh. (Southern KSA) ❧ Place butter and outer peelings of pomegranate on burns. (Southern KSA)

Diabetes: Mix 1 tablespoon of myrrh, 1 cup of cress, $1/2$ cup black seed, $1/2$ cup ground pomegranate, 1 cup dried, ground cabbage root, and a small spoon of cumin seeds with yogurt (to make it easier to eat) and eat it on an empty stomach. This is good for diabetes. (Eastern KSA)

Heart Trouble: Soak a lot of black seed in water, drink the water and eat the seeds. Also, drink soaked pomegranate in boiled water and a spoon of honey. (Eastern KSA)

Sinus Congestion: Cut up pomegranate peelings into smallish pieces and boil. Take some of the boiled liquid, after it has cooled, in a cupped hand and 'toss' it up the nostrils. It will clear up the sinuses quickly. (Eastern KSA)

Skin Care: For healthy skin, our mothers used to use the soaked skin of pomegranate to wash our faces and hands. (Eastern KSA)

Stomach Complaints: Use pomegranate peelings for the stomach (antiseptic). (Central KSA)

Stomach Ulcers: Mix pomegranate peelings with honey and eat the mixture. (Eastern KSA) ❧ For ulcers of the stomach, use this for a month or until you recover: Crush dried pomegranate peelings until they become powder. Mix with an equal amount of honey. Eat a teaspoon of the mixture first thing in the morning before eating. (Central KSA)

Dried pomegranate peelings.

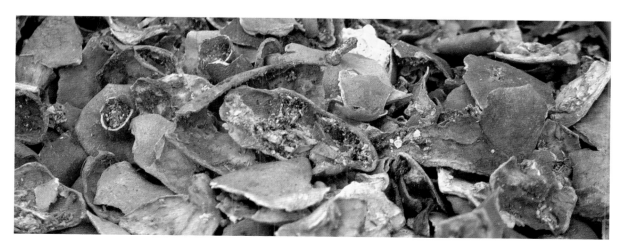

RESEARCH

Pomegranate peelings have been found to have antioxidant activity in various lab experiments involving rats. (Chidambara Murthy, K.N., et al. 'Studies on antioxidant activity of pomegranate (Punica granatum) peel extract using in vivo models.' *J Agric Food Chem.* 2002 Aug 14;50 (17): 4791-5.)

The latest research shows that topical application of pomegranate fruit extract to mouse skin significantly inhibits development of skin cancer. (Afaq, F., et al. 'Pomegranate Fruit Extract is a Novel Agent for Cancer Chemoprevention: Studies in Mouse Skin (Abstract 1547). 'American Association for Cancer Research Annual Conference, Oct. 26-30, 2003.)

Recent research provides evidence that pomegranate may have a positive effect against human breast cancer. (Kim, N.D., et al. 'Chemopreventive and adjuvant therapeutic potential of pomegranate (Punica granatum) for human breast cancer.' *Breast Cancer Res Treat.* 2002 Feb; 71(3): 203-17.)

DID YOU KNOW?

🐝 Pomegranate tree flowers are a pretty red colour. Male and female flowers grow on the same plant. The smaller male flowers fade and fall off after blooming. Female flowers become fruit and ripen 5-7 months after flowering. Trees are productive for at least 30 years.

🐝 Pomegranate seeds are rich in vitamin C and are a good source of dietary fibre.

🐝 Commercially produced pomegranate syrup is called grenadine.

🐝 The Prophet Muhammad suggested soothing, almost spiritual, properties of this fruit when he said, 'Eat the pomegranate, for it purges the system of envy and hatred.'

🐝 The Romans called the pomegranate fruit *punicum*, the Latin name for Carthage, because they believed that the best pomegranates came from there.

🐝 The Spanish name for the pomegranate is *granada*, and its fruit appears on Granada's city seal.

🐝 In India, pomegranate is used in a traditional Ayurvedic remedy for dysentery. It is also useful in gargles and is said to ease fevers and assist in counteracting diarrhoea.

🐝 For centuries, the pomegranate has played a role in Cyprus marriage rituals. In some parts of the island, pomegranate seeds are thrown at newlyweds as they exit the church. In others, a pomegranate is smashed in the path of the couple or against the front wall of their future home. These practices are to wish love and fertility to the newlyweds.

🐝 Pomegranate is believed to be the inspiration for the hand-tossed explosive called a grenade. When a pomegranate is dropped on a hard surface, it bursts and seeds are tossed everywhere. The military borrowed the modern French name for the fruit, *grenade*.

🐝 *King's American Dispensatory* (1898) describes the pomegranate as 'one of the oldest of drugs, having been used from time immemorial.' It also cites the rind and the bark of pomegranate as specific remedies for tapeworm infestation.

PURSLANE

Portulaca oleracea (Wild Purslane)

Portulaca oleracea var. sativa (Kitchen Garden
   Purslane)

Portulacaceae Family

Arabic: *barbeer, barbir, rijlah, baql hamqa', baglah*

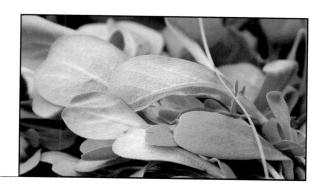

Purslane is a warm-climate annual with fleshy green leaves similar to cress. It grows wild in dry soils, but a kitchen variety, *Portulaca oleracea var. sativa*, is cultivated as a vegetable crop.

   In Arabia, kitchen purslane is available year-round in modern grocery stores as well as at the outdoor vegetable markets. It is used as a salad herb, a vegetable and a kitchen remedy. It is often cooked with meat or grain.

HOW TO USE

1. Chop leaves into a green salad.

2. Use sprigs of purslane as a garnish.

IN THE KITCHEN

Store in the refrigerator. When purchased fresh, purslane lasts for about a week. It can be stewed with meat or chicken.

FAMILY REMEDIES ACROSS ARABIA

Warts: Rub the leaves of *rijlah (P. oleracea v. sativa)* on warts to treat them. Then, when dry, rub with black seed oil. (Eastern KSA)

RECIPE | Fattoush, p. 185

DID YOU KNOW?

🐛 The 1st-century Greek pharmacologist Dioscorides used purslane to fight fevers and treat ailments of the stomach and bladder.

🐛 The Arab physician al-Kindi used purslane, along with other simples, to treat pustules on the lips. He prescribed purslane seeds in medicines for coughs and sore throats, and as an ingredient in a mouthwash.

🐛 *Portulaca oleracea* grows in Sudan, where the whole young plant is used for food and for treating abdominal disorders.

RESEARCH

Jordanian researchers report that a crude extract of purslane accelerates the wound-healing process by decreasing the surface area of the wound and increasing the tensile strength. (Rashed, A.N., et al. 'Simple evaluation of the wound healing activity of a crude extract of *Portulaca oleracea* L. (growing in Jordan) in *Mus musculus* JVI-1.')

A research team of the United Arab Emirates' Ministry of Health has confirmed claims of traditional medicine that kitchen-variety purslane *(var. sativa)* has a role in relief of pain and inflammation. The team found that an extract of dried leaves and stems showed significant anti-inflammatory and analgesic activity. (Chan, K., et al. 'The analgesic and anti-inflammatory effects of *Portulaca oleracea* L. subsp. *Sativa* (Haw.) Celak.' J Ethnopharmacol. 2000 Dec; 73(3): 445-51.)

ROSE

Rosa damascena

Rosaceae (Rose) Family

Arabic: *ward*

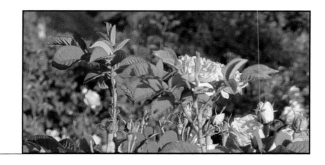

In Saudi Arabia, the mountain resort city of Taif is famous for its fragrant Damask roses and for production of rose water and attar, the essential oil made from the petals of the rose. Rose water and attar are very popular at celebrations, such as the two *Eid* holidays, weddings and other special occasions.

In earlier days, petals were collected and transported by camel caravans to Makkah, where specialists of Indian origin distilled them into attar. Then, about 200 years ago, the manufacture of Damask rose oil became more efficient when distillers brought this art to Taif. Today there are hundreds of farms which cultivate the rose and approximately 60 distillation plants. The most famous rose-growing areas in Taif are al-Hada and al-Shafa.

The best time to harvest rose petals is early in the morning before sunrise. Flowers should be picked before they are affected by the sun's rays and processed immediately after picking because much of the oil, contained mostly in the petals, evaporates if flowers are left for more than a few hours. This is critical for maintaining the high quality fragrance of the attar.

Al-Qadhi Rose Factory, Taif, Saudi Arabia.

HOW TO USE

1. Add rose water to special dishes when cooking.

2. Apply to face with a cotton pad for cosmetic use as an astringent.

IN THE KITCHEN

Rose water provides subtle flavour in cooking, especially in desserts. Rose water is also added to tea.

Rose petal harvesters can get SR25 (US$6.70) for 1,000 petals. This is usually a day's pay. It takes 25,000 petals to make 100 grammes of oil. This is why 1 gramme of oil can cost SR20,000-25,000 (US$5,300-$6,700).

RESEARCH

Damask rose essential oil has demonstrated antimicrobial activity against Staph bacteria *(Staphylococcus aureus)*. (Aridogan, B.C., et al. 'Antimicrobial activity and chemical composition of some essential oils.' *Arch Pharm Res.* 2002 Dec; 25(6): 860-4.)

Rosa damascena's anti-infective and anti-inflammatory properties contribute to the effectiveness of a certain brand of therapeutic eyedrops, researchers report. (Biswas, N.R., et al. 'Evaluation of Ophthacare eye drops – a herbal formulation in the management of various ophthalmic disorders.' *Phytother Res.* 2001 Nov; 15(7): 618-20.)

FAMILY REMEDIES ACROSS ARABIA

Rose water is a traditional remedy for the heart and the stomach.

Childbirth: Use cinnamon and a natural mixture of flowers (roses). (Southern KSA)

Eye Care: Dissolve barley sugar in rose water with saffron and use this liquid to bathe the eyes to ease a stye. (UAE)

Flatulence (Intestinal Gas): Roses dispel gases in the stomach, as do thyme and lavender. (Northern KSA)

Heart Trouble: Use rose water. (Central KSA)

Insomnia: Drink rose water with sugar if you have trouble sleeping. (UAE)

Skin Care: Clean the skin and face with rose water or flower water. (Central KSA) ❧ Grandmother used a corn flour mask with rose water, which was applied on the face until it dried and then washed off. (Eastern KSA)

DID YOU KNOW?

❧ The Damask rose is an ancient, fertile hybrid from Western Asia. Its origins are somewhat disputed, but most experts believe it is a cross between Europe's *Rosa gallica* and either the Levant's *Rosa phoenicia* or India's *Rosa moschata*.

❧ A tale regarding the origin of the Damask rose in Taif relates that a lone traveller from India brought the rose to this mountainous region hundreds of years ago. Another story says that it was a pilgrim from the ancient rose plantations of Persia. A third idea is that the Ottoman Turks, who occupied the Hejaz in the 16th century, brought the roses.

❧ Taif, in the mountains of Saudi Arabia's Western Province, produces vegetable, cereal and orchard crops, in addition to the rose. Abundant harvests include the fig, apricot, lime, pomegranate and almond. Taif is the summer residence of the Saudi Royal Family and a refuge from coastal humidity and desert heat.

❧ Cooked flower heads, the yield of the distillation process, are sold to local cattle farmers in Arabia who feed them to their cows. Farmers are rewarded with a mildly rose-flavoured milk.

❧ Ninth-century physician Hunain ibn Ishaq used the seed, oil and aqueous solution of rose in medicines for treatment of eye diseases.

❧ Al-Kindi, author of a 9th-century medical formulary, prescribed rose oil for treatment of haemorrhoids, ulcers and boils, and used rose petals in poultices for the stomach, liver and spleen, and in medicines for sore throat and mouth ailments.

SAFFRON

Crocus sativus
Iridaceae (Iris) Family
Arabic: *za'faran, za'fran*

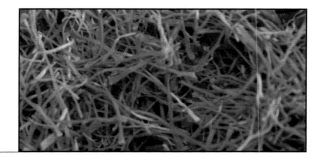

Native to the Middle East, saffron was introduced to Europe by the Moors (the Muslim Arabs and Berbers of northwest Africa) who conquered most of Spain in the 8th century. From Spain, or al-Andalus as the Arabs called it, saffron was carried to Italy and France, where it became popular. Although not completely new to the British Isles, saffron was brought back to England by the crusaders of the 13th century. Historically, saffron has been used for medicine, perfume, dye and as a cooking spice.

Saffron refers to the dried, red stigmas collected from the flowers of *Crocus sativus*. Its high price is better understood when we learn that some 75,000 flowers are required to make one pound of dried saffron. Commercial producers of saffron today include Spain, Iran and India.

HOW TO USE

The dried red stigmas produce a bright yellow or orange colour when added to water. If a recipe requires ground saffron, one can crush or grind it to a powder. Be sure it is evenly distributed when added to the recipe. Sifting the ground saffron with the dry ingredients is one way to insure a good mix.

If using whole saffron threads, soak them for about 10 minutes in a warm liquid required by the recipe, such as milk, water or broth. The colour and flavour of the stigmas will be released into the liquid. A pinch of saffron to a cup of liquid yields enough colour and flavour for about one pound or one-half kilo of rice. A little saffron goes a long way.

IN THE KITCHEN

Saffron can add taste and colour to breads, chicken and rice dishes. Spanish paella, for example, derives its yellow colour from saffron.

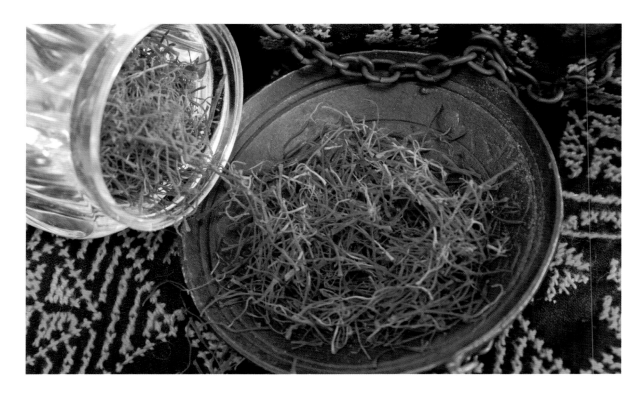

FAMILY REMEDIES ACROSS ARABIA

Headaches: Drink peppermint, saffron, ginger and water. (Southern KSA)

Heart Trouble: We use soaked saffron. We put water in a glass, then add a little saffron and drink. (Eastern KSA)

Skin Care: My mother put saffron on her lips and cheeks. (Central KSA) ❧ My grandmother used saffron with safflowers. She mixed them with water. She put them on her face like a mask. (Central KSA)

RESEARCH

Saffron extract and its main constituents, the carotenoids, possess antitumour effects and chemopreventive properties against cancer, according to a growing body of research. (Abdullaev, F.I. 'Cancer chemopreventive and tumoricidal properties of saffron (*Crocus sativus L.*).' *Exp Biol Med (Maywood)*. 2002 Jan; 227(1): 20-5.)

Saffron has been shown to have a positive effect on learning and memory in experimental animals, suggesting it may be useful for treating neurodegenerative disorders accompanying memory impairment. (Abe, K., and H. Sato. 'Effects of saffron extract and its constituent crocin on learning behaviour and long-term potentiation.' *Phytother Res*. 2000 May; 14(3): 149-52.)

DID YOU KNOW?

❧ Comparing the beauty of his beloved to a garden, Solomon (Chapter 4 verse 14 of *Solomon's Song* in the Old Testament) lists saffron, cinnamon, frankincense and myrrh as some of the plants cultivated in this metaphor. We sense the magnitude of his admiration because these plant products commanded very high prices in ancient markets.

❧ Today saffron remains the most expensive spice in the entire world.

❧ Scholars studying frescoes at Thera, a Greek island in the Aegean, believe the wall paintings (dating from 1500 or 1600 BC) depict a goddess presiding over the manufacture and use of a drug from the saffron flower. This suggests saffron has been used as a medicine for at least 3,500 years.

❧ The ancient Greeks believed that saffron originated in Asia Minor, but it appears to have been first cultivated in Crete. The Romans regarded saffron as a curative and an aphrodisiac, and would sprinkle it on the marriage bed.

❧ The celebrated physician-philosopher al-Kindi used saffron in a wide range of medications, including a nasal medicine for scrofula, and medicines for a swollen head, swollen liver, sore throat, bad teeth and gums, eye disease, epilepsy and insanity. He also used it in a stomachic and in a drug to purify the air and prevent the spread of epidemics.

❧ The 13th-century English scientist Roger Bacon believed saffron would delay ageing and add joy to life.

❧ Spain and Iran are the world's biggest producers of saffron, accounting together for more than 80 per cent of global production. Spanish saffron is widely regarded as the world's finest.

SAGE

Salvia officinalis
Lamiaceae (Mint) Family
Arabic: *maryamiya, maramiya*
Other English: Kitchen Sage, Garden Sage

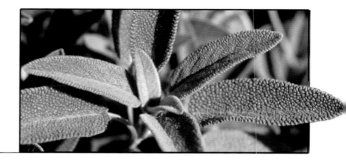

Why should a man die while sage grows in the garden?
— Medieval saying

In the Middle East, sage is valued for its medicinal properties. Huge bags of light gray-green dried sage leaves are displayed and available for purchase in traditional outdoor markets as well as in the super-markets and herb shops.

In addition to its medicinal role, sage is also used as a spice in Arabic cooking, including in marinades for kebabs and some meat dishes. But its culinary role is not as extensive in Arabia as it is in the Mediterranean, where sage is a common ingredient in Spanish, Italian and Greek dishes.

HOW TO USE

1. Use the leaves fresh or dried.

2. Infuse the leaves to make a tea.

IN THE KITCHEN

Adding a little honey helps to reduce the slightly bitter taste of sage tea.

DID YOU KNOW?

☙ *Salvia officinalis,* a fragrant perennial, is sometimes called garden or kitchen sage to distinguish it from wild sage or sagebrush, an artemisia that also has medicinal uses.

☙ The genus name Salvia comes from the Latin term *salvere*, meaning 'to be in good health.'

☙ Sage originated in the Mediterranean and Asia Minor, and today is perhaps most popular in Italy. There are also several New World species of sage, including pineapple sage *(Salvia rutilans).*

☙ The ancient Romans used sage to treat epilepsy, snake bites and lung disorders. Pliny the Elder asserted that the fragrance of sage would cleanse the air.

☙ Sage is linked by ancient legend to the Virgin Mary, and is said to derive its medicinal healing powers from her. This may explain the Arabic name for the herb, *maryamiya*, which means 'Marian [herb (*'ushba*)],' i.e., an herb pertaining to Mary. The mother of Jesus holds a place of honour in Islam.

☙ A species of sage that grows in Iran and Afghanistan, *Salvia macrosiphon*, locally called *kanocha* or *marv*, is used in traditional medicine there. Its mucilaginous seeds are prescribed for debility, and are used to treat heart disturbances in pregnancy and phlegmasia (internal inflammation) after childbirth.

FAMILY REMEDIES ACROSS ARABIA

Sage leaves are antiseptic and make an excellent gargle for sore throats. Sage is known to aid poor digestion and irregular periods.

Abdominal Pain: Sage is for stomach problems, abdominal pains, colon problems and gas. (Eastern KSA) ❧ The leaves are dried, boiled, then strained and the liquid is taken to treat the abdomen. (Eastern KSA) ❧ Take peppermint and sage for abdominal pain. (Southern KSA) ❧ Boil sage with tea to reduce abdominal pains. (Southern KSA)

Childbirth: To strengthen a mother after childbirth, use fenugreek, cress, cinnamon, sage and peppermint. (Eastern KSA)

Flatulence (Intestinal Gas): Boil sage and let sit for 10 minutes after turning off the fire. This is for stomachaches and stomach gases. (Central KSA)

Insomnia (Trouble Sleeping): Take peppermint, lemon and sage. (Eastern KSA)

Menstrual Pain: For menstrual periods, boil sage with cinnamon. (Western KSA) ❧ Peppermint, cinnamon, chamomile and sage are taken for menstrual cramps. (Eastern KSA) ❧ Cinnamon helps the blood flow. Sage strengthens the womb. (Western KSA) ❧ Use cinnamon and ginger. Boil together for 25 minutes, then drink. Or use sage. (Central KSA) ❧ For menstrual cramps, steep herbs such as cinnamon and/or sage to make tea. (Bahrain)

Overweight: Sage is taken for pains and to lose weight. (Northern KSA)

Sore Throats: For a sore throat, take boiled sage. (Western KSA)

Stomachache: Use fenugreek, cress, cinnamon, peppermint and sage. (Eastern KSA) ❧ Use sage and peppermint for stomachaches. (Southern KSA)

RESEARCH

Sage is known to possess compounds with antioxidant properties, such as carnosic acid, carnosol, rosmanol and caffeic acid. (Matsingou, T.C., et al. 'Antioxidant activity of organic extracts from aqueous infusions of sage.' *J Agric Food Chem.* 2003 Nov 5; 51(23): 6696-701.)

German researchers have found certain substances in sage, such as caffeic acid and salvianolic acids, to be effective against the Leishmania parasite and some pathological viruses without damaging host cells. (Radtke, O.A., et al. 'Evaluation of sage phenolics for their antileishmanial activity and modulatory effects on interleukin-6, interferon and tumour necrosis factor-alpha-release in RAW 264.7 cells.' *Z Naturforsch* [C]. 2003 May-Jun; 58(5-6): 395-400.)

SAMH

Mesembryanthemum forsskalei
Aizoaceae Family
Arabic: *samh, ghasul*

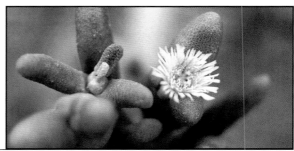

Finnish explorer Georg Wallin, travelling through north-west Arabia in 1845, came across an unusual pod-plant in the desert called *samh*. In pods the size of an ordinary pea, the plant produces a large number of tiny reddish seeds, prized and collected by the local Bedouins. To obtain the seeds, Wallin recommends soaking the harvested pods in water. They will open and the seeds will drop to the bottom, while the pods float to the surface. *Samh* is not cultivated; it is harvested wild in July. Traditionally, Bedouin men, women and children of all ages take part in the harvesting.

Samh grows in the Sinai Peninsula (notably along the eastern bank of the Suez Canal) and in the northern Arabian desert, particularly in the Tabarjal area of the al-Jawf region, i.e., in the dunes of the Nafud desert. A small succulent 'iceplant' less than 25 cm high, with bright yellow flowers, it thrives in areas characterized by sandy plains or slopes, low rainfall and high temperatures. *Samh* plants also favour low salinity.

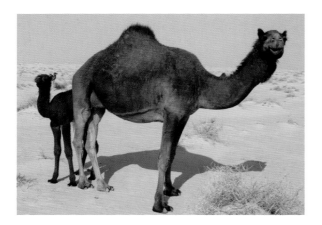

HOW TO USE

1. Gather the seeds and dry them in the sun.

2. Grind the seeds coarsely or into a finer flour for use in baking.

3. Boil the seeds with mashed dates.

IN THE KITCHEN

Samh seeds can be ground into flour and baked into bread. Wallin describes the bread loaves as 'reddish,' good-tasting and (for him) somewhat indigestible. British explorer Charles Doughty, who visited the area some three decades after Wallin, tasted *samh* 'wild-bread' at Maan, and described it as 'black and bitter, but afterward I thought it sweet-meat, in the further desert of Arabia.'

Samh seeds can be coarsely ground in a hand mill, mixed with water and then cooked into a porridge. William Palgrave, another English explorer, was served *samh* porridge while visiting Northern Arabia in 1862. He said it looked 'much like a bowl full of coarse red paste, or bran mixed with ochre.' One of Palgrave's Bedouin companions described the porridge as 'not so good as wheat, and rather better than barley-meal.' Charles Doughty thought *samh* porridge was 'good' and tasted 'as camel milk' – perhaps because some had been added to his bowl.

The roasted or raw seeds, as well as the flour, can be kneaded with butter into a mass of pitted dates, and rolled into balls to be eaten while travelling. Doughty thought this made for 'a very pleasant and wholesome diet for travellers.' Czech explorer Alois Musil sampled this foodstuff at al-Jawf in the 1920s and said he thought it tasted like chocolate.

FAMILY REMEDIES ACROSS ARABIA

Samh seeds are valued for their nutrition. They are very high in protein, amino acids and other nutrients and can be used to counter malnutrition in times of famine or scarce resources.

DID YOU KNOW?

⸏ Bedouins told explorer Wallin that *samh* grows only in a limited range of the northern desert of Arabia, near al-Jawf, and only in places where rain has fallen during the time of the Pleiades. This was the time of year when the Pleiades constellation rises above the horizon just after sunset. According to Arabian tradition, the rains that come during this time bring an abundance of plant life, including *samh*.

⸏ Botanist James P. Mandaville says that among the Shammar tribesmen of Northern Saudi Arabia, the best sort of *samh* is called *hurr* ('pure'). An inferior type grows around Baq'a and Kafhah in the same area.

⸏ In the 19th century, *samh* flour from al-Jawf was marketed in the Najd region, where it was considered a delicacy.

⸏ Wallin reported that *samh* thrived in the lands of the Sherarat Bedouins, but he observed that these tribesmen 'are not fond of it, and exchange it in great quantities with the villagers for other food.' Palgrave, two decades later, saw things differently – he described *samh* as an important staple of the Sherarat Bedouin diet.

⸏ Another species of the same plant family, reportedly with similar qualities, is found at Muweileh, and is called *da'ā*, according to Wallin. Musil calls this plant *du'ā*, a name recorded by Mandaville for *Aizoon canariense*. The U.S. Food and Drug Administration labels *A. canariense* as toxic and includes it in the Poisonous Plant Database.

RESEARCH

Scientists at the College of Agricultural and Food Sciences of King Faisal University in al-Hasa have conducted studies of Saudi *samh* seeds and found that they have 'high nutritional potential.' The seeds have a very high protein content, in excess of 22%. (Jasser, M.S., et al. 'Studies on *samh* seeds. *(Mesembryanthemum forsskalei* Hochst) growing in Saudi Arabia: 2: Chemical composition and microflora of *samh* seeds.' *Plant Foods Hum Nutr.* 1995 Oct; 48(3):185-92.)

The ground seeds were found to make a successful, nutritious substitute for wheat flour in bread and cookies. (Mustafa, A.I., et al. 'Studies on samh seeds *(Mesembryanthemum forsskalei* Hochst) growing in Saudi Arabia: 3. Utilization of *samh* seeds in bakery products.' *Plant Foods Hum Nutr.* 1995 Dec; 48(4):279-86.)

Ground *samh* seeds have also been studied – somewhat inconclusively – for possible use as a non-meat high-protein extender in beef (hamburger) patties. (Elgasim, E.A., and M.S. Al-Wesali. 'Water activity and Hunter colour values of beef patties extended with *Samh (Mesembryanthemum forsskalei* Hochst) flour.' *Food Chemistry* 69 (2000) 181-85.)

SARCOCOL

Astragalus sarcocolla
Fabaceae (Bean) Family
Arabic: *anzarut, kuhl farsi*
Other English: Sarcocolla

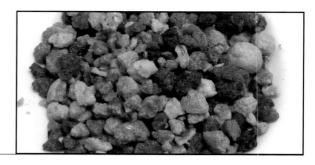

Sarcocol, known to the Arabs as *anzarut* or *kuhl farsi* (Persian kohl), is a frankincense-like gum resin from a perennial shrub originating in Kurdish areas of Iran. It has a long history of medicinal use from the Mediterranean area to the Himalayas.

Anzarut is closely related to a number of other gum-producing Astragalus species, including *A. gummifer*, the source of the common food additive gum tragacanth, a thickening agent.

Families from Tabuk and Hail in northern Saudi Arabia have reported using *anzarut* for home remedies. Inhabitants of the Eastern Province use it as well.

HOW TO USE

Crush to a powder for topical application or for blending with oil or various dry substances. It may also be taken internally.

IN THE KITCHEN

Sarcocolla is a mixture of small yellowish, reddish or brownish agglutinate masses. When heated, it emits an odour similar to heated sugar. It is initially sweet but has a bitter aftertaste. Its taste has been compared to that of licorice root.

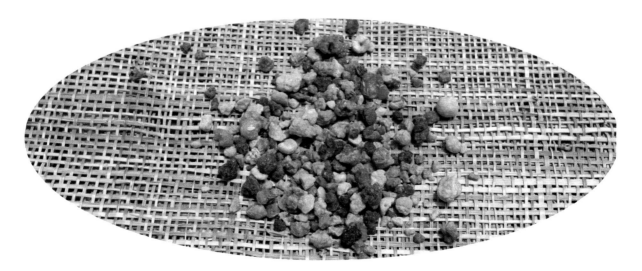

RESEARCH

A cousin of the sarcocol plant, astragalus root *(Astragalus membranaceus)* is used extensively in Chinese traditional medicine, and has been shown in tests to strengthen the human immune system. (Chu, D.T., et al. 'Immunotherapy with Chinese medicinal herbs II. Reversal of cyclophosphamide-induced immune suppression by administration of fractionated *Astragalus membranaceus* in vivo.' *Journal of Clinical Laboratory Immunology*, 1988, 25:125–9.)

FAMILY REMEDIES ACROSS ARABIA

A traditional remedy, it is still used in eastern Saudi Arabia and other parts of the Middle East for healing wounds and treating skin disorders. Sarcocol is also taken internally as a digestive and for other purposes.

Cuts or Other Flesh Wounds: *Anzarut* is used to treat cuts or other flesh wounds. (Eastern KSA)

Indigestion: Take *anzarut*. (Northern KSA)

Newborn Care: *Anzarut*, *shabba* and myrrh (mixed) and kohl are used on babies. (Northern KSA) ⚘ Crush to a powder and mix with oil. Gently rub the mixture onto the soft part of the skull of a newborn baby. (Eastern KSA) ⚘ Use black seed and *anzarut*. (Northern KSA)

DID YOU KNOW?

⚘ The Graeco-Roman physician Galen said sarcocol was used for healing and cicatrizing wounds (i.e., creating scar tissue to heal wounds). The name 'sarcocol' or 'sarcocolla' comes from the Greek words for 'flesh glue.'

⚘ Hunayn ibn Ishaq (809-877 AD), in his textbook on ophthalmology, includes sarcocol in a prescription of mixed powders to sharpen vision, prevent eye itching and treat various other eye problems.

⚘ Spanish pharmacologist Ibn Biklarish (12th century) and Saladin's court physician Maimonides (13th century) also mention sarcocol as a remedy for eye problems.

⚘ In the *Complete Herbal* of 17th-century English physician Nicolas Culpeper, sarcocol is mentioned as an ingredient in making pills.

⚘ Al-Kindi used sarcocol as a salve to remove black spots from the skin, in prescriptions for leprosy and abscesses, and for cataracts.

⚘ Dr I.E.T. Aitchison, a British army surgeon who explored Iran and neighbouring regions in the 19th century, reported that Muslim women of the area used sarcocol to improve their appearance and make their skin glossy.

⚘ In India, Parsi healers have long used sarcocol in a plaster for broken bones. The gum is also applied to the face and ears to ease neuralgic pain.

⚘ In traditional Tibetan medicine, the gum of *Astragalus sarcocolla* is used as a mild laxative.

⚘ The name sarcocolla is also applied to the gum of several species of Penaea (particularly *P. sarcocolla* and *P. mucronata*), which grow in central and southern Africa and have similar properties to *Astragalus sarcocolla*. This African version of sarcocolla has been used in the treatment of wounds, ear discharges and scrofula.

SIDR

Zizyphus spina-christi
Rhamnaceae (Buckthorn) Family
Arabic: *sidr, sidra*
Other English: Lote-tree, Christ's Thorn

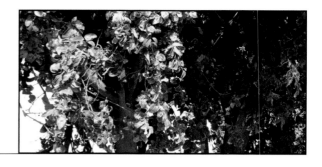

The hardy lote-tree is a true Arabian native species. A wild, thorny and shrubby tree, it grows in low areas where ground water accumulates.

The Qur'an mentions the *Sidr* tree on three occasions: as a thornless tree in paradise (56: 28), as a wild and useless tree when thorny (34: 16) and as a landmark of heavenly knowledge (53: 14-16).

The powdered dried leaves of this precious tree have long been used in Islam to wash the bodies of the dead in preparation for burial. Its dried and powdered leaves are also mixed with water and applied by women as a hair wash. This *sidr* paste is reputed to soften hair and strengthen the roots.

HOW TO USE

1. Dry the leaves.

2. Grind the dried leaves into powder.

IN THE KITCHEN

The cultivated *sidr* tree bears edible fruit – called *nabaq* or *nabiq* in many parts of Arabia, and *kenar* in the Western Province – which is still sold in the more traditional markets.

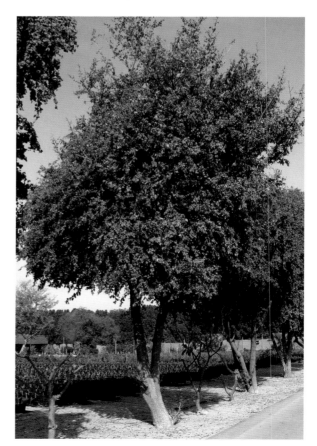

Saudi Aramco Nursery, Dhahran, Saudi Arabia.

RESEARCH

The aqueous extract of *Z. spina-christi* root bark may have sedative activity. (Adzu, B., et al. 'Effect of Zizyphus spina-christi Wild aqueous extract on the central nervous system in mice.' *J. Ethnopharmacology.* 2002;79:13-6.)

Researchers in Egypt have investigated the leaves, fruits and seeds of *Zizyphus spina-christi* for antiviral, antifungal and antibacterial properties, and have identified a number of flavonoids, including such virus-killers as quertecin and hyperoside. (Shahat, A.A., et al. 'Chemical and biological investigations on *Zizyphus spina-christi* L.' *Phytother Res.* 2001 Nov;15(7):593-7.)

FAMILY REMEDIES ACROSS ARABIA

Mary Beardwood, in *The Children's Encyclopaedia of Arabia*, reports on the varied uses of the *sidr* tree: the seeds are powdered with lemon juice to treat liver complaints, the roots are used for arthritis and rheumatism, the fruits are used for bronchitis and coughs. It is also used to treat dandruff, reduce weight and cleanse the body. *Sidr* is a stomachic, appetizer and astringent.

Hair Care: Mix enough hot water with one-half cup of *sidr* leaf powder to form a paste. Apply by rubbing the paste into the hair. Rinse and repeat. (KSA) ᔐ Grind *sidr* leaves and add to water. After soaking 10 minutes, wash hair with the mixture and comb. When applied a second time, do not rinse; simply comb hair thoroughly. (Southern KSA) ᔐ After soaking *sidr*, it is put on wet hair and combed well. Then it's left, but not to dry. Rinse later with water. (Southern KSA) ᔐ Use *sidr* to wash the hair and make it smooth and silky. (Eastern KSA)

Hair Loss: For hair loss, use *sidr* and henna. (Southern KSA) ᔐ Use olive oil and *sidr*. (Western KSA) ᔐ Use henna water and *sidr* water. (Northern KSA)

Hygiene: Use *sidr* leaves for washing instead of soap by grinding the leaves and mixing with water. (Southern KSA) ᔐ Apply *sidr* to your body. Then using a loofah, treat it like shower gel. (Western KSA) ᔐ Wash with *sidr* and *shabba* (alum). (Eastern KSA)

DID YOU KNOW?

ᔐ *Zizyphus spina-christi* is reputed to be the source of Jesus Christ's crown of thorns. This popular Middle Eastern legend is repeated among Muslims, and is cited in notes to Abdullah Yusuf Ali's translation of the Qur'an.

ᔐ J.R. Rodwell, another Qur'an translator, recounts a legend that a lote-tree grows in Heaven, beside the throne of God, whose many leaves are inscribed with the names of all living persons. This tree is shaken on the night of the 15th of Ramadan each year, and those leaves that fall foretell the passing of all those fated to die in the coming year. Says Arabian specialist James P. Mandaville: 'The story appears to have no basis in orthodox Islam and is not generally current in Arabia today.'

ᔐ The *sidr* or *nabaq* tree grows in Yemen, and for many centuries its wood was used for windows and doors in traditional buildings in cities like Shibam, home of the towering mud-brick buildings dubbed the 'world's first skyscrapers'.

ᔐ Yemeni *sidr* merchant Abdu Ali Naji reports receiving the herb from local Yemeni harvesters as well as from suppliers in Wadi al-Dawaser, al-Hasa, Medina, and Riyadh in Saudi Arabia. (*Riyadh Daily*, Nov. 4, 1996)

ᔐ In western Sudan, the fruit of the *sidr* tree is considered a delicacy. The bitter-sweet pulp of the fruit is also dried and milled to produce flour.

TARTHUTH

Cynomorium coccineum

Cynomoriaceae Family

Arabic: *tarthuth, turthuth*

Other English: Maltese Mushroom, Malta Fungus, Desert Thumb, Red Thumb

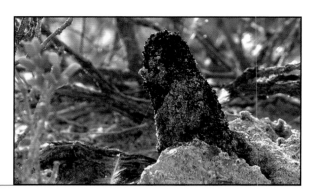

Seated on the slope of a dune, Mahmoud watches his father's camels grazing on the spring foliage. It has been a long morning, and he now awaits the return of his father's white pickup truck. Suddenly he spies a burst of burgundy colour against the tan of the sands and the pale green of the spring growth. Beside a saltbush he sees four little dark-red clubs poking up from the sand. *Tarthuth!* Mahmoud is hungry and thirsty, and nature has furnished him with one of its tastiest snacks.

He brushes the sand from the base of one of the stalks and cuts it off at the root with his pocket knife. The pungent smell makes him grin. Mahmoud cuts away the reddish skin – tightly coated with tiny button flowers – and exposes the succulent white flesh beneath. He slices off a wet piece and pops it in his mouth. Sweet and juicy, refreshing, like ripe fruit ... As he chews, contentment passes over him.

Mahmoud is lucky: *tarthuth* emerges from the sands for only a brief period each year, after the winter rains. Finishing his snack, he cuts off the remaining red clubs to take back to his family.

The people of eastern Saudi Arabia have been harvesting *tarthuth* for thousands of years. This curious parasitic plant, which draws nutrients from the roots of saltbushes, has long pleased the palates of passing Bedouins and their camels, filled grocers' baskets in local markets, and served as survival food in times of dire famine.

Tarthuth also has a long history as a medicinal herb in the Middle East and the Mediterranean region.

HOW TO USE

1. When harvesting, cut the stalks at ground level or below.

2. Wash the stalks, peel with a knife and slice like a carrot.

3. Dry the stalks and grind into powder.

4. Steep the powder of dried *tarthuth* to make a medicinal tea.

IN THE KITCHEN

The succulent, astringent flesh should be eaten as soon as possible after harvesting, before the sweetness fades and a mild bitterness sets in.

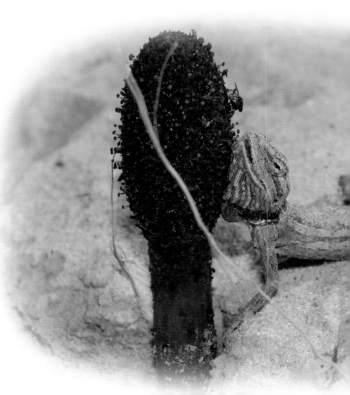

FAMILY REMEDIES ACROSS ARABIA

Bleeding: Apply to wounds like a poultice to stop bleeding. (Eastern KSA)

Ulcers and Other Stomach Ailments: Eat a few fresh slices of *tarthuth* or sip some tea brewed with the powdered stalk. (Eastern KSA)

DID YOU KNOW?

☙ *Cynomorium coccineum* grows in dry coastal areas in a swath of countries from Spain to Iran. Its stalks bloom in early spring, after the winter rains. It is well known in eastern Saudi Arabia and adjacent Gulf states.

☙ The ancient Hebrews ate *tarthuth* as a famine food. In the *Book of Job* (30:4), starving Israelites survive on a plant sometimes translated as 'juniper root' – modern botanists argue this is *C. coccineum,* and not the inedible root of the juniper bush.

☙ Arab physicians of the Middle Ages called *tarthuth* 'the treasure of drugs' because of its many pharmaceutical uses, particularly as a remedy for blood disorders, gastro-intestinal ailments and reproductive problems, including infertility and impotence. It was reputed to be an aphrodisiac.

☙ Al-Kindi (800-870) used *tarthuth* as a salve for foreign material under the skin that causes acute itching. Another famed Arab physician, Al-Razi (865-925), recommended tarthuth for nasal, uterine and anal haemorrhage.

☙ In the 17th century, the Knights of Malta jealously guarded and harvested *tarthuth* (or 'Maltese Mushroom') crops on a tiny island of the Malta chain called Fungus Rock. They used the herb to heal wounds, dysentery, ulcers, haemorrhages and venereal disease, among other ailments. The Knights' Grand Master sent Maltese Mushroom as a special gift to the crowned heads of Europe.

☙ *Tarthuth* has a Far Eastern cousin, *C. songaricum* or *suo yang.* Its brownish spikes have long been considered an effective medicinal agent in Chinese medicine, treating kidney problems, intestinal ailments and impotence.

RESEARCH

Scientists at King Saud University's College of Agricultural and Veterinary Medicine found that extracts of *Cynomorium coccineum,* administered orally, had significant positive effects on the reproductive development and fertility of male and female rats. (Abdel-Magied, E.M., et al. 'The effect of aqueous extracts of *Cynomorium coccineum* and *Withania somnifera* on testicular development in immature Wistar rats.' J *Ethnopharmacol* 2001 Apr; 75(1): 1-4; Al-Qarawi, A.A., et al. 'The effect of extracts of *Cynomorium coccineum* and *Withania somnifera* on gonadotrophins and ovarian follicles of immature Wistar rats.' *Phytother Res* 2000 Jun; 14(4): 288-90; and Abd el-Rahman, H.A., et al. 'The effect of the aqueous extract of *Cynomorium coccineum* on the epididymal sperm pattern of the rat.' *Phytother Res* 1999 May; 13(3): 248-50.)

In 1978, researchers in Iran reported that the fresh juice of *Cynomorium coccineum* was 'found to possess significant blood pressure lowering activity' in testing on dogs. (Ikram, M., et al. 'Hypotensive agent from *Cynomorium coccineum.*' *Pahlavi Med J* 1978 Apr; 9(2): 167-81.)

THYME
Thymus vulgaris
Lamiaceae (Mint) Family
Arabic: *za'tar, sa'tar, hasha'*

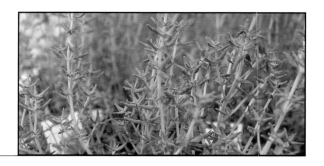

When dining in the Middle East, many enjoy dipping bread in olive oil and then in *za'tar* for a delicious taste. Although *za'tar* is the word for 'thyme' in the Arabic language, it is also a term for a Middle Eastern spice blend of powdered dried thyme, sumac, and sesame seeds. Each region makes *za'tar* a little differently. Syrian *za'tar* is considered one of the best.

The term *za'tar* is also used for wild thyme, *Thymus serpyllum*, a similar, more robustly flavoured, species that grows in Iran and Kurdistan.

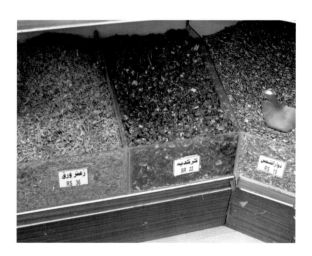

HOW TO USE

1. Use fresh green thyme leaves when called for in recipes.

2. Use dried thyme leaves as part of the aromatic spice blend called *za'tar*.

3. Sprinkle *za'tar* (fresh thyme or the spice blend) on meatballs or vegetables.

4. Use the *za'tar* spice blend with olive oil as a dip for bread.

IN THE KITCHEN

Pita bread rounds topped with *za'tar* alone or with melted cheese or *labna* are indescribably delicious. It is easy to make your own blend of *za'tar* or buy it ready-made in a Middle Eastern food store.

Store *za'tar* in an airtight container away from direct light.

Herb display in Jeddah, Saudi Arabia.

RESEARCH

Thyme's essential oils show significant antibacterial activity. The most effective is the oil from thyme in full flower. (Marino, M., et al. 'Antimicrobial activity of the essential oils of *Thymus vulgaris* L. measured using a bioimpedometric method.' *J Food Prot.* 1999 Sep; 62(9): 1017-23.)

In one experiment, 52 different plant oils and extracts were investigated for activity against 10 microbes. Thyme oil was found to be the most effective against *Candida albicans* and *E. coli.* (Hammer, K.A., et al. 'Antimicrobial activity of essential oils and other plant extracts.' *J Appl Microbiol.* 1999 Jun; 86(6): 985-90.)

FAMILY REMEDIES ACROSS ARABIA

A general remedy for colds, flu, fevers, coughs and bronchitis is to drink 4-5 cups of thyme tea a day. Thyme is antiseptic, antispasmodic and antifungal. It is also an expectorant and vermifuge (worm expeller).

Colds and Coughs: Thyme is for coughs. (Northern KSA) ❧ Thyme is eaten or mixed with hot water for colds and abdominal pains. Put a tablespoon in a glass of hot water. (Eastern KSA) ❧ For coughs and colds, use *za'tar* with hot water, as well as myrrh and honey. (Western KSA) ❧ Thyme boiled with water and sugar helps to relieve coughs. (UAE)

Diarrhoea: Thyme leaves stop diarrhea. (Eastern KSA)

Fatigue: Grind radish seeds in onion juice with powdered thyme and eat the mixture with olive oil and cheese to strengthen the body. (Eastern KSA)

Flatulence (Intestinal Gas): Use thyme and lavender. (Northern KSA)

Indigestion: Eat onion with date, fennel, black seed, thyme and cheese for indigestion. (Eastern KSA)

Liver : Thyme cleans the liver and abdomen. (Northern KSA)

Memory: Thyme softens the throat and is useful for memory. (Central KSA)

Stomach Pain: Boil dried thyme leaves in water, then strain and drink for stomach pain. (Eastern KSA) ❧ Use thyme and myrrh. (Eastern KSA)

DID YOU KNOW?

☙ Five millennia ago, the Sumerians used thyme as an antiseptic.

☙ The ancient Egyptians employed thyme as an ingredient in the mummification process.

☙ The Arab philosopher-scientist al-Kindi (800-870 AD) used thyme in a medicine to treat a bacterial infection or rash called St Anthony's Fire (erysipelas).

☙ The Islamic physician al-Razi (865-925 AD) regarded thyme as an appetite enhancer, stomach purifier and treatment for flatulence.

☙ Thyme is traditionally regarded as tonic, carminative, emmenagogue and antispasmodic. The oil has long been used in the West as a local application for neuralgic and rheumatic pains.

☙ Thyme is widely grown commercially for its leaves and essential oils.

☙ Thyme is one of a small number of herbs that have more flavour dried than fresh. Others are rosemary and oregano.

TRUFFLES, DESERT

Terfezia spp and *Tirmania spp.*
Terfeziaceae Family
Arabic: *faga', fuga', faz', kamah, kam'a chim'a,
terfex, terfax*

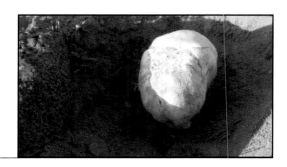

In March 1908, thanks to a winter of helpful rains, the desert truffles *(faga')* were plump and plentiful in the deserts of al-Wudijan west of Baghdad. Prince an-Nuri ibn Shaalan of the powerful Rwala Bedouin tribe had encamped there, and one of his men, Miz'el, was busy searching and digging, in hopes of finding enough of the underground delicacies to make a respectable campfire dinner.

As the Czech explorer Alois Musil relates it: 'He had gathered his mantle full of them ... and in the evening presented them to an-Nuri, who gave one to each person present. Together they roasted them over the fire; even the Prince himself had fetched some butter, crumbled into it the baked truffles, and eaten them with relish.'

Desert truffles are a type of globular underground mushroom that attaches itself to the roots of plants, akin to the celebrated forest truffles of Europe. Both types resist cultivation, and usually grow only in the wild. The desert truffle (either the *Terfezia* or *Tirmania genus*) has a milder flavour than its European cousin, *Tuber spp.*

Desert truffles can be found in arid, sandy areas around the Mediterranean, particularly in North Africa, and across the great deserts of Syria, Iraq and Saudi Arabia. In Morocco they are known as *terfez* (probably the source of the Latin name), in western Egypt *terfas*, in Syria and Iraq *kam'a*, in southern Iraq *cham'a* and in Saudi Arabia and the Gulf *faga'*.

Unlike their European counterparts, desert truffles do not require trained dogs or pigs to locate them. The fungal fruits develop close to the surface, forming distinctive mounds of cracked soil. In eastern Saudi Arabia, Bedouins searching for *faga'* after the winter

---

HOW TO USE

Desert truffles are cooked in various dishes. Wash the truffles very carefully to remove sand. Peel and slice them.

IN THE KITCHEN

White truffles *(Tirmania nivea)* are said to be the most delicious. Faga' can be boiled in water or milk, roasted or sautéed. They should only be cooked for a few minutes. Sautée them in butter or, if camping, roast them in campfire ashes. Bahrainis sometimes prepare truffles with rice.

---

rains know they will often find them growing in association with several species of Helianthemum, known locally as *rugrug*.

Ancient legends in the Middle East associate truffles with thunderstorms. Some believe the truffles' size and numbers are influenced by the intensity of the thunder. Whether or not this is true, scientists say desert truffle yields are definitely related to total rainfall and its distribution during the winter rainy season. However, a good desert truffle harvest can result from as little as 200-250 mm of rain in a season, provided there is good rain before the second week of December.

Desert truffles come in various colours. North African *terfez* are often white. Kuwaiti truffles are frequently pale brown. Saudi *faga'* range from white to red to brown to black.

Says Saudi writer Ni'mah I. Nawwab: 'Desert truffles, *faq'*, have their aficionados in Najd, as elsewhere, and during the spring, especially after it rains, families often go truffle hunting. According to a lady from 'Unayzah, 'it requires extremely good eyesight as well as experience to spot the slightly raised and cracked spots that indicate that truffles are growing underneath.' When the expedition returns laden with truffles, women get the job of cleaning them. The truffles are often 'very sandy, and removing their outer skin is a long job,' she adds. However, truffle-lovers say it's worth it, particularly when they taste them in soups, gravies and rice. Truffles continue to be included in traditional dishes such as *tharid* and *ruzz mutabbaq*, a layered rice dish in which they are prepared with meat or chicken and vegetables.' ('The Culinary Kingdom,' *Aramco World*, January/February 1999)

| RECIPE | Faga' Mahmoose (Sautéed Truffles), p. 193 |

RESEARCH

Spanish researchers have determined that raw desert truffles (*Terfezia claveryi*) and certain other fungi have stronger antioxidant properties than four common food antioxidants, including alpha-tocopherol [E-307]. (Murcia, M.A., et al. 'Antioxidant activity of edible fungi (truffles and mushrooms): losses during industrial processing.' *J Food Prot.* 2002 Oct; 65(10): 1614-22.)

In a study at King Faisal Specialist Hospital in Riyadh, investigators found that an ethanol extract of *faga'* (*Tirmania pinoyi*), when combined with two known carcinogens, inhibited cell mutations induced by the carcinogens. (Hannan, M.A., et al. 'Mutagenic and antimutagenic factor(s) extracted from a desert mushroom using different solvents.' *Mutagenesis.* 1989 Mar; 4(2): 111-4.)

FAMILY REMEDIES ACROSS ARABIA

Truffles offer extra nutritional value. These desert fungi are regarded by some Bedouins as a substitute for meat. *Terfezia claveryi* samples from Saudi Arabia have been shown to contain 16 per cent protein, 28 per cent carbohydrates, 4 per cent fibre and 2 per cent fat. The samples were rich in minerals. They also contained nine saturated and four unsaturated fatty acids and 29 amino acids.

DID YOU KNOW?

🐾 In Saudi Arabia, the larger Middle East and Arab North Africa, desert truffles have been collected as a delicacy since ancient times.

🐾 Cairo's Fatimid rulers feasted on desert truffles collected in the Muqattam Hills to the east of the city. In the 19th century, 'truffles were sold in such quantities in Cairo's souks that far from being choice dainties they had become cheap and common,' said historian Edward Lane.

🐾 Street vendors in Baghdad used to – and may still – sell egg and desert-truffle sandwiches (wrapped in pita bread) to hungry passersby.

🐾 Desert truffles are a valuable resource for villagers in Turkey's Anatolia region, according to the Food and Agriculture Organization. The truffles (*Terfezia boudieri*) are harvested in spring and summer. Most are consumed in village households and the rest are sold to local traders both in fresh and dried form.

🐾 Gazelles have been seen digging up truffles from beneath the desert sand and eating them with great pleasure, Bedouins told explorer Alois Musil.

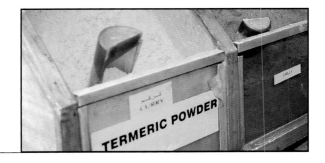

TURMERIC

Curcuma longa, C. domestica
Zingiberaceae (Ginger) Family
Arabic: *kurkum*

India, the world's largest supplier of turmeric, is geographically close to the Arabian Peninsula, and perhaps that explains the popularity of turmeric in Saudi Arabia and neighbouring countries.

In ancient times, Omani sailors played an important role in developing the Indian Ocean sea trade, which greatly contributed to the prosperity of South Arabian culture and the variety of goods which found their way to the peninsula. Ancient traders planned their trading schedules based on wind patterns, travelling to India with the summer monsoon winds blowing from the southeast and returning home with the winter monsoon winds blowing north-west. Waiting for shifts in the wind allowed them time to unload their goods and then load their ships again with items of trade.

Often called 'Indian saffron,' the turmeric rhizome was one of the ancient trade products brought by sea from India. Today turmeric is widely used as a spice, cosmetic and dyestuff, and remains part of traditional medicine from Egypt to Iran.

HOW TO USE

1 Slice, grate, chop or grind turmeric to a paste with other ingredients. Then, use it as you would fresh ginger root.

2 Grind dried turmeric into powder.

3 Use whole pieces of dried turmeric in pickling.

IN THE KITCHEN

Slicing a piece of turmeric rhizome reveals the deep yellow colour used to brighten curry powders and a variety of foods. When colouring rice dishes, it is also sometimes a substitute for saffron. Turmeric is mixed with other spices and used in such dishes as *kabsa, matazeez* and *jarish*.

It is easier to buy ready-ground turmeric rather than grinding it yourself. To maintain a fresh supply, buy powdered turmeric in small quantities and store it in an airtight container away from strong light.

Wear rubber gloves when handling fresh turmeric to avoid staining your hands.

RECIPE	*Chicken Kabsa, p. 190*

RESEARCH

Curcuma, a yellow pigment in turmeric root *(C. longa)*, exhibits anti-inflammatory, antitumour and antioxidative properties, and is currently being studied for its possible use in human cancer prevention and treatment, as well as in cardiovascular and cholesterol therapy. (Baatout, S., et al. 'Effect of *curcuma* on radiation-induced apoptosis in human cancer cells.' *Int J Oncol.* 2004 Feb; 24(2): 321-9; Miquel, J., et al. 'The *curcuma* antioxidants: pharmacological effects and prospects for future clinical use. A review.' *Arch Gerontol Geriatr.* 2002 Feb; 34(1): 37-46.)

FAMILY REMEDIES ACROSS ARABIA

Burns: Apply ash and turmeric. (Northern KSA)

Childbirth: To strengthen a mother after childbirth, use fresh soup as a meal. It's good for the woman after delivery. It consists of fresh meat, chopped onion and a spice mixture of black pepper, turmeric and cumin. Boil these ingredients until the meat is ready to eat. Serve it to the mother. (Southern KSA)

Colds and Coughs: Burn turmeric sticks and inhale the fumes to cure coughs. (UAE) ♣ Use honey with turmeric (*kurkum*) for colds or coughs. (UAE)

Cuts: Apply turmeric and coffee. (Eastern KSA)

Eyes: To treat opaque corneas, grind some turmeric very fine, add a little water, strain it through a fine cloth, and then drip it into the eye. (Soqotra Island, Yemen)

Infections: If the infection shows signs of redness and pus, clean the site with a strong salt water solution, and then smear it with a paste of turmeric and water, or dust it with turmeric powder. (Socotra, Yemen)

Skin Ailments: For multiple sores, grind together some salt and turmeric and apply to the sores each day until they clear up. (Socotra, Yemen) ♣ A mixture of salt, dates and turmeric powder is used to heal bruises. (UAE)

DID YOU KNOW?

♣ Turmeric is cultivated in rocky soil in Indonesia, China, India and Bangladesh. The underground stem or rhizome is the most used part.

♣ In traditional Chinese medicine, turmeric has been used to control blood clotting and haemorrhage.

♣ In India, turmeric is used to treat diarrhoea, urinary tract infections, conjunctivitis, sore throats and other ailments.

♣ In Indian cuisine, turmeric is an ingredient of virtually all curry powders.

♣ Because turmeric is an edible colouring, the food industry uses it to colour mustard, butter, cheese, and liqueurs.

♣ Turmeric is used to dye cotton and silk.

♣ Al-Kindi (800-870 AD) used turmeric in a medicine for throat and mouth pustules, and in a dentifrice to strengthen the gums.

♣ The US Patent and Trademark Office in 2001 rejected six attempts to patent the medicinal properties of turmeric. The office said turmeric is a centuries-old Indian discovery and cannot be patented.

WALNUT BARK

Juglans spp.
Juglandaceae (Walnut) Family
Arabic: *deerum*

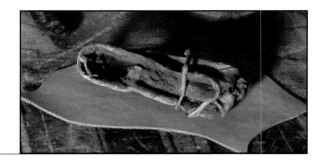

A container filled with thin bark strips folded up and tied into bundles is one of the interesting curiosities at traditional Arabian markets. This product is called *deerum* in Arabic and is the bark of the walnut tree.

Although not widely used nowadays, *deerum* is a reminder of the traditional self-reliance and ingenuity of peoples in the Arabian Peninsula during times of more limited resources.

HOW TO USE

1. Chew the end of the bark until soft.

2. Rub the bark vigorously on lips for a natural dark brown lipstick.

3. Use the bark as a toothbrush to clean teeth and gums.

IN THE KITCHEN

You may wish to rinse this bark off with water or clean with a damp cloth before using it because it gets quite dusty in the marketplace.

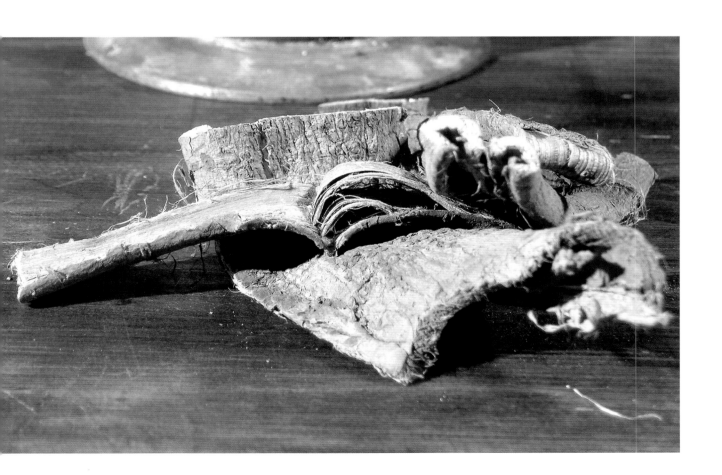

FAMILY REMEDIES ACROSS ARABIA

The bark of the walnut tree is astringent and cleansing. It strengthens the gums and acts as an anti-inflammatory. It has been used to treat gum disease.

Oral Care: *Deerum* is for the lips. *Deerum* is a stick that cleans teeth and puts dark brown colour on the lips. (Northern KSA) ❧ *Deerum* is for whitening the teeth and for treating gum inflammation. (KSA)

RESEARCH

Researchers at King Faisal University's College of Medicine in Dammam, Saudi Arabia, have found broad-spectrum antimicrobial activity (against staph and strep bacteria, *E. coli* and *Candida albicans*, among other pathogens) in an extract made from the bark of common walnut (*Juglans regia*). They noted that 'brushing the teeth with this bark may improve oral hygiene, prevent plaque and caries formation, and reduce the incidence of gingival and periodontal infections.' (Alkhawajah, A.M. 'Studies on the antimicrobial activity of *juglans regia*.' *Am J Chin Med.* 1997; 25(2): 175-80.)

Researchers in India reported anticancer properties in a number of medicinal plants, including the bark powder of *Juglans regia*. (Arora, S., et al. 'Indian medicinal plants as a reservoir of protective phytochemicals.' *Teratog Carcinog Mutagen.* 2003; Suppl 1: 295-300.)

DID YOU KNOW?

❧ Walnut is the common name for about 20 species of deciduous trees in the walnut family, *Juglandaceae*.

❧ Pliny the Elder, author of the Roman encyclopedia *Natural History*, reported that walnut trees were introduced into Italy from Persia. Roman writer Varro, born in 116 BC, noted that walnut was growing in Italy during his lifetime.

❧ Walnut bark is a traditional source of yellow-brown dye.

❧ Herbalist Maud Grieve, in *A Modern Herbal* (1931), states that walnut bark, dried, powdered and made into a strong infusion, is a useful purgative.

❧ Walnuts are rich in protein and high in potassium and other minerals such as zinc and iron.

❧ Walnut bark has been added to the bath for treatment of rheumatism as well as sore and aching muscles and joints.

❧ Walnut bark tincture, in a little carrier oil (sweet almond, jojoba, etc.) has been used to treat swellings and skin problems, and to encourage healing.

❧ In the late 1800s, the US National Eclectic Medical Association, a group of medical doctors who favoured botanical medicine, recommended the bark of the black walnut, *Juglans nigra*, as a topical treatment for ringworm and other skin diseases.

WORMWOOD (a)

Artemisia herba-alba or *Artemisia sieberi*
Asteraceae (Aster) Family
Arabic: *sheeh, shih, qaysum, gharira*
Other English: Armenian Wormwood,
    Desert Wormwood, White Artemisia,
    White Mugwort

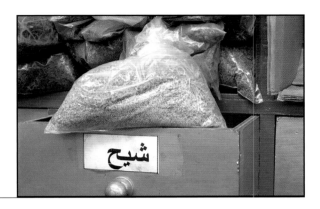

Sheeh is one of the most intensely aromatic of all plant species in Northern Arabia. The fragrance of its crushed foliage is lemony and sweet, and more intense than that of its sister species *Artemisia judaica,* also sometimes called *sheeh.* Armenian wormwood is found in the northern plains near Hafr al-Batn and in Summan, in the northeast corner of the peninsula. It is also found in the northwest, notably amid the granite peaks of Saudi Arabia's Hisma mountain range and its Jordanian extension, the Shera mountains.

Finnish explorer Georg A. Wallin, on his way into Arabia a century and a half ago, was captivated by the herbal aromas of the Shera region, which were dominated by the scent of *sheeh*: '... [T]he wild vegetation is luxuriant and varied, and the valleys and hills abound in good pasture-grounds, where, among the most varied desert-plants, the species of wormwood – so much prized by the Bedawies, and so much celebrated by ancient poets under its still current name of *Shîh* – grows in the greatest abundance. The pure atmosphere on the lofty mountains, refreshed as it is by the strong odour of aromatic herbs, makes the air of Sherâ one of the best and most salubrious I ever breathed, and highly invigorates the originally strong and healthy constitution of the inhabitants.'

Sheeh has traditionally been used for stomach and intestinal ailments as well as diabetes. Among the Bedouins of the North, it is also used as a smoke inhalant. According to Czech explorer Alois Musil, Bedouins used *sheeh* smoke to treat the infectious bacterial disease glanders in horses and to exorcise animals believed to be possessed by evil jinn.

HOW TO USE

1. Dry the leaves and grind them into powder.

2. Crumble dried leaves and smoke them in a pipe.

3. Infuse the leaves or powder to make a tea.

IN THE KITCHEN

Fresh leaves of *sheeh* can be boiled along with vegetables to add a sour taste. Use small amounts.

RESEARCH

Artemisia herba-alba extract is attributed with 'considerable lowering of elevated blood sugar' in patients with diabetes mellitus, and 14 out of 15 patients had 'good remission' of diabetic symptoms – without side effects. (Al-Waili, N.S. 'Treatment of diabetes mellitus by *Artemisia herba-alba* extract: preliminary study.' *Clin Exp Pharmacol Physiol* (1986 Jul) 13(7):569-73.)

Diabetic rabbits, given an oral extract of *A. herba-alba*, showed a marked decline in blood sugar levels. (Twaij, H.A., and A.A. Al-Badr. 'Hypoglycemic activity of *Artemisia herba alba*.' *J Ethnopharmacol* (1988 Dec) 24(2-3):123-6.)

An aqueous extract of *Artemisia sieberi* was one of the top six anti-cancer agents identified among 66 desert plant extracts tested on cultured melanoma cells. (Sathiyamoorthy, P., et al. 'Screening for Cytotoxic and Antimalarial Activities in Desert Plants of the Negev and Bedouin Market Plant Products.' *Pharmaceutical Biology.* Jul 99, Vol. 37, Issue 3, p. 188-95.)

FAMILY REMEDIES ACROSS ARABIA

Childbirth: Use *al-ghar* [bay leaf], *sheeh* [wormwood] and rose water. (Western KSA) ❧ Eat *marquq* (a broth dish with whole-wheat pasta), milk, fenugreek, *aseeda* (gruel), *sheeh*, cumin, thyme and *qaysoom (Achillea fragrantissima)*. (Northern KSA)

Diabetes: Drink a tea made from *sheeh* 2-3 times a day. (KSA and Bahrain)

Indigestion: Take *sheeh* and lemon. (Northern KSA)

Kidneys: For kidney problems or heat in the urine, make a tea from *sheeh*. Bring 100 ml of water to a boil and pour over 10 grams of *sheeh*. Do not boil *sheeh* in water. Drink tea 2-3 times a day. (Central KSA and Bahrain)

Stomachache: Use *sheeh*, lemon and chamomile. (Northern KSA) ❧ For bulging stomachs, gases and stomach complaints in general, boil leaves and drink. Drink *sheeh* cold or warm. (Northern KSA)

Weakness: Use *sheeh* leaves for paleness and dizziness. (Northern KSA)

DID YOU KNOW?

❧ *Artemisia herba-alba* has been widely used in Iraqi folk medicine for the treatment of diabetes.

❧ *A. herba-alba* is widely popular in North African countries as a remedy for skin problems, including abscesses, herpes lesions and acne. The dried powdered leaves are used for healing wounds and burns.

❧ *Sheeh*, sold under the name of *Barbary santonica*, is used from Morocco to Egypt as an anthelmintic, to expel parasitic intestinal worms.

❧ The *sheeh* plant is popularly known as *diqn al-shaikh* (old man's beard) in Sudan, where its leaves are used to remedy abdominal colic, kidney pain, indigestion, gonorrhoea, flatulence, diabetes, irregular periods, gum problems and other ailments.

❧ Al-Kindi, in his 9th-century *Medical Formulary*, lists burnt Armenian wormwood (*shih*) as an ingredient in a medicinal tooth powder that polishes teeth, removes decay, treats bad breath and generally protects the mouth.

❧ Arabian explorer Sir Richard F. Burton recommended pillows stuffed with wormwood for insomnia.

❧ *Artemisia herba-alba* is a known abortifacient. Its use should be avoided during pregnancy.

WORMWOOD (b)

Artemisia judaica
Asteraceae (Aster) Family
Arabic: *bu'aythiran, ubaithran, sheeh*
Other English: Judean Wormwood,
Biblical Wormwood

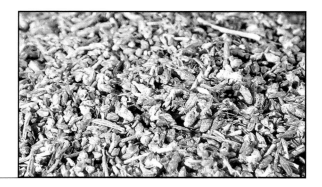

Bu'aythiran is the Arabic name for this northwestern Arabian species of Artemisia.

Professor Michael Zohary, who taught botany in Jerusalem for many years, describes *Artemisia judaica* as a handsome, strongly fragrant dwarf shrub with comparatively large heads of foliage, and one of the leading perennials of the desert.

Botanist Ahmad Migahid of King Saud University, in his book *Flora of Saudi Arabia*, reports that *bu'aythiran* is a local name applied to three different plant species: *Artemisia judaica*, *Achillea fragrantissima*, and *Teucrium polium*.

HOW TO USE

1. Dry the leaves and grind them into powder.

2. Crumble dried leaves and smoke them in a pipe.

3. Infuse the leaves or powder to make a tea.

IN THE KITCHEN

Arabian explorer Alois Musil (1868-1944) reported that Shammar Bedouin mixed dates with chopped *bu'aythiran (Artemisia judaica)* to flavour and preserve them. They boiled the mixture until the liquid evaporated. The resulting foodstuff kept well during long journeys.

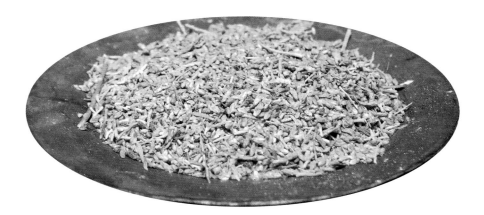

RESEARCH

The essential oil of *Artemisia judaica* gathered in Southern Sinai has been shown to inhibit the growth of various bacteria and other microorganisms. (Al-Gaby, Ali M., and Reda F. Allam. 'Chemical Analysis, Antimicrobial Activity, and the Essential Oils from Some Wild Herbs in Egypt'. *Journal of Herbs, Spices & Medicinal Plants*. Vol. 7, No. 1, 2000.)

FAMILY REMEDIES ACROSS ARABIA

Insomnia: Stuff a pillow with *bu'aythiran*; the pleasant fragrance helps you sleep. (Northern KSA)

Repellant: Because of its distinctive aroma, branches and twigs of *bu'aythiran* are wrapped with stored clothes to protect them from moths. (KSA) ❧ Leaves and twigs are kept in the mattress and blankets to repel dangerous or bothersome insects such as scorpions and bugs. (KSA)

Rheumatism: Smoke the dried leaves of *bu'aythiran* in a pipe as medicine for rheumatism. (KSA)

Skin Care: Use *bu'aythiran* for beautiful, healthy skin. (Northern KSA)

Stomachache: Brew a tea and drink to relieve a stomachache. (KSA)

DID YOU KNOW?

❧ *Artemisia judaica* was probably the wormwood of the Old Testament, the herb that bittered the waters in the desert during the ancient Hebrews' wanderings. Its leaves give off a pungent odor when disturbed or crushed, and have an extremely bitter taste.

❧ In the Old Testament, calamities and sorrows have metaphorically been linked to noxious and bitter herbs, such as wormwood. (Deuteronomy 29:18; Jeremiah 9:15; 23:15; Lamentations 3:15,19; Amos 5:7; Revelations 8:10-11)

❧ *Artemisia* has been used as a beverage and as a medicine. In ancient times, the herb was steeped in wine to counteract the effect of alcohol.

❧ Assyrian herbalists of old used *artemisia* as an expectorant.

❧ Al-Samarqandi, a 13th-century physician in Afghanistan, prescribes *Artemisia judaica* for treatment of swellings and bruises.

❧ *Artemisia* shrubs are herbaceous perennials and provide valuable colour and form in the herb garden.

❧ *Bu'aythiran* is sometimes used as a name for *Achillea fragrantissima*, which is more commonly called *qaysum*.

YARROW

Achillea fragrantissima
Asteraceae (Aster) Family
Arabic: *qaysum, qeesum, gesoom, qaysum jabali, bu'aythiran, baatharaan*
Other English: Fragrant Desert Yarrow, Lavender Cotton, Milfoil

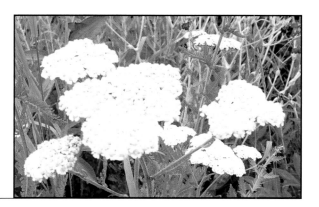

The pump station and town of al-Qaysumah, located on the Trans-Arabian Pipeline (Tapline) in northern Saudi Arabia, take their names from this fragrant perennial.

A wooly, erect herb that grows up to one metre tall, *qaysum* is distributed in the Najd and in the northern and eastern regions of the Arabian Peninsula.

Its leaves and twigs are kept in mattresses and blankets to repel insects. They are also placed with stored clothing to protect against moths.

HOW TO USE

Use the dried leaves or flowers to make a tea.

IN THE KITCHEN

Qaysum is added to food to strengthen a mother, especially during the 40 days following childbirth.

Qaysum leaves can be dried and used with regular tea as a flavour enhancement or brewed alone to make tea.

DID YOU KNOW?

❧ The Asteraceae family, which includes daisies, dandelions and thistles, was formerly known as the Compositae family.

❧ *Achillea fragrantissima* is used in some parts of the Eastern Mediterranean to treat hypoglycaemia and diabetes.

❧ In the Middle Ages, leading Arab physicians like Ibn al-Azraq (d. 890) and al-Suwaydi (600-690) prescribed the milk of camels fed on *Achillea fragrantissima* to correct digestive disorders, detoxify the liver and treat hepatitis.

❧ Traditional medicine in Jordan prescribes *qaysum*, prepared as a decoction and taken orally, to stop uterine bleeding.

❧ In Northern Arabia, aromatic pillows stuffed with *Achillea fragrantissima* are sometimes given as wedding gifts.

❧ Southernwood (*Artemisia arborescens*) shares the Arabic name *qaysum*. This plant is well-liked by camels in the desert.

FAMILY REMEDIES ACROSS ARABIA

The Bedouin use the leaves and flowers in an infusion for the treatment of coughs. In Arabian medicine, *qaysum* is regarded as a carminative, stomachic, anti-spasmodic, febrifuge, anthelmintic, diuretic and cholagogue. It is also used traditionally in Saudi Arabia as an anti-inflammatory to treat rheumatism, arthritis and other similar ailments.

Coughs: Use the flowers to make a tea. (KSA)

Childbirth: To strengthen a mother after childbirth, eat *marquq* (a broth dish with whole-wheat pasta), milk, fenugreek, gruel *(aseeda)*, *sheeh*, cumin, thyme and *qaysum*. (Northern KSA)

Stomachaches : Use *qaysum* leaves. (Northern KSA)

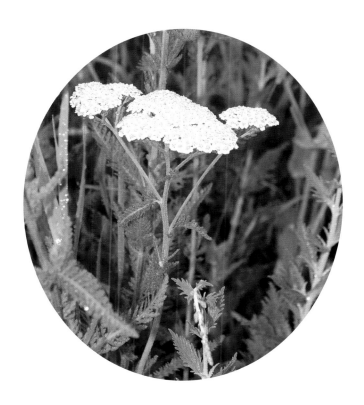

RESEARCH

An aqueous extract of *Achillea fragrantissima* was one of the top three anti-cancer agents identified among 66 desert plant extracts tested on cultured melanoma cells. (Sathiyamoorthy, P., et al. 'Screening for Cytotoxic and Antimalarial Activities in Desert Plants of the Negev and Bedouin Market Plant Products.' *Pharmaceutical Biology*. Jul 99, Vol. 37, Issue 3, p. 188-95.)

Essential oil from *A. fragrantissima* has been shown to kill certain bacteria, including the yeast *Candida albicans*. (Barel, S., et al. 'The antimicrobial activity of the essential oil from *Achillea fragrantissima*.' *J Ethnopharmacol*. 1991 May-Jun; 33(1-2): 187-91.)

OTHER
NATURAL REMEDIES

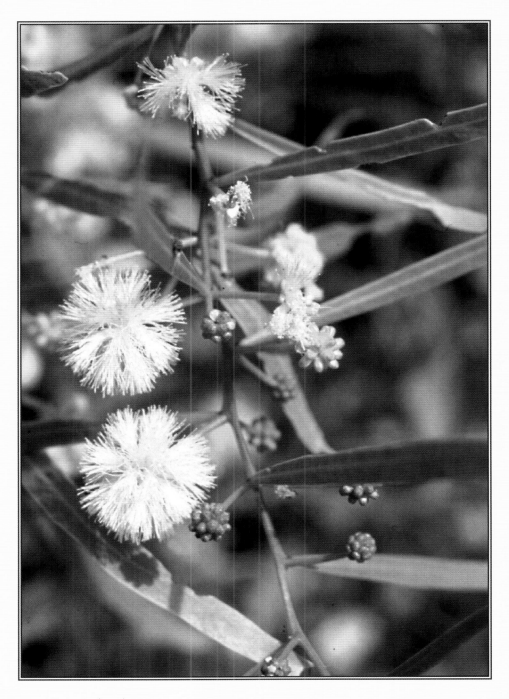

Acacia gerrardii subsp.

ACACIA

Acacia gerrardii subsp. Negevensis; A. iraqensis, A. nilotica
Arabic: *talh, sammara, sillima, siala, garat*

A common Arabian tree, usually with distinct trunk, 3-10 m high. This is one of two large-trunked acacias, the other being *A. raddiana*, that are known in the vernacular as *talh* and that are important constituents of the woody vegetation along wadis of the Tuwayq uplands in central Arabia. Mandaville believes it might be a rather copious producer of gum arabic *(al-samgh al-'Arabi)*, although he found no exploitation of this product in the Eastern Province. He reports collecting 'large tears of fine, clear, light amber, tasteless gum from what appeared to be this species in Wadi Hanifah, Najd.'

In the United Arab Emirates, the seeds of a sister species, *A. nilotica* (locally called *garat*), are ground into a powder to dry out second-degree burns. Al-Kindi used acacia for lesions and for dentifrices, and used gum arabic in cough and eye medications. Acacia was employed to strengthen eyelashes and eye muscles. The seed of acacia is today used in tanneries and in a medicine for diarrhoea. The gum is an astringent and emollient. It is used internally for ulcers and spitting of blood, and externally in collyria. According to Doughty: 'Clear gum arabic drops are distilled upon the small boughs [of a solitary acacia tree near Ethlib]; that which oozes from the old stock is pitchy black, bitter to the taste, and they say medicinal: with this are caulked the Arab coasting hoys which are built at Wejh.' This specific tree was said to be possessed by jinn.

APPLE OF SODOM

Calotropis procera
Arabic: *'ushar*
Other English: Sodom Apple

A plant of the Milkweed family, whose pear-shaped fruit and latex have medicinal properties. Found in eastern, central and northwestern Saudi Arabia as well as in Bahrain. The raw latex is often considered poisonous, but reports of its toxicity may be exaggerated, according to Mandaville. (A powerful cardiac poison known as gigantin is derived from a related species, *Pergularia giganta*, in India.) The Bedouins of eastern Arabia do regard the plant as poisonous and their livestock are said to keep away from it. But the Bedouins sometimes use small quantities of the latex for medicinal purposes.

A Bani Hajir elder told Mandaville that a safe, effective dose could be obtained by scooping out the seeds and pulp from a halved ripe fruit and drinking sheep, goat or camel milk from the remaining green skin 'cup'. According to Doughty, 'the country people gather the sap and sell it for a medicine to the Persian pilgrims.' In the United Arab Emirates, the bitter sap was traditionally dried and used to fill aching tooth cavities. Poultices made from the leaves were placed over joints to heal rheumatism. Levey identifies the Sodom apple with *Ladanum asclepiad*, which al-Kindi used in a dentifrice, for lengthening the hair, and in a formula for exterminating worms and purifying the air during an epidemic.

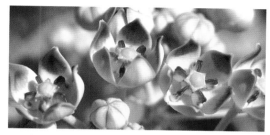

Apple of Sodom

BLACK NIGHTSHADE

Solanum nigrum
Arabic: *shajarat al-bulbul* ('Nightingale bush' in Qatif, referring to the birds' apparent
   fondness for the berries – Mandaville), *ruzbaraj* (Persian-origin name, meaning 'fox
grapes'), *'inab al-tha'lab* ('fox grapes'), *muqnin* (Levey)
Other English: Garden Nightshade, Petty Morel

The medicinal value of Black Nightshade is linked to its belladonna-like alkaloids. Black nightshade is sometimes called poisonous, but Mandaville reports seeing farmers in Qatif in eastern Saudi Arabia pluck the ripe black berries and eat them raw, laughing at the notion they might be poisonous. Local birds also eat the fruit. Mandaville suggests that the plant's content of the toxic alkaloid solanine might vary depending upon the variety and environment, and warns against eating the berries in any quantity. Krueger reports that the foliage is poisonous but the berries edible. The plant is a common weed in Iraq and Iran. Women place the seeds on their cheeks to remove freckles and aid the complexion. In Egypt and North Africa, the plant is used only externally for inflammation, tumours and haemorrhoids.

Al-Kindi used black nightshade in an ointment taken nasally, as a liver medicine, an oral medicine and a haemorrhoid treatment, and a sedative narcotic, as well as in an application for erysipelas. Avicenna also used black nightshade in some of his preparations.

BLOND PSYLLIUM

Plantago ovata
Arabic: *qurayta'*
Other English: Ispaghula

One of the numerous plantain species used medicinally. Its pink or gray-brown seeds contain a significant amount of mucilage, which swells in the intestines, acting as a bulk laxative and soothing irritated membranes. Saudi Bedouins were reported earlier in this century to use the seeds of blond psyllium as a laxative.

Across the Gulf in Iran, Baluchistan and northern India, the seeds are given for gonorrhea and used as a diuretic.

CAPER

Capparis spinosa
Arabic: *shafallah, kabbar*

A prickly shrub whose flower buds and berries are pickled for use in sauces and other recipes. Pickled capers have been used as a condiment initially in the Mediterranean area and now worldwide over the past 2,000 years. Called *kabbar* in early Arabia, the common caper plant's root bark was used in a poultice for spleen problems and haemorrhoids, and its leaves were used in a drug for spirits, according to al-Kindi. Today the bark, which has a bitter taste, is used in central Saudi Arabia for treating arthritis. A tea can be made from the plant, which works as an emetic and is used to treat indurations and scrofula as well as disorders of the liver and spleen.

CARALLUMA

Caralluma quadrangula
Arabic: *dij'* (Oman), *shereyon* (Dhofar)

A strange-looking member of the Milkweed family, this plant, when not flowering, can easily be mistaken for stone. It is gray, leafless, with succulent stems that are roughly square in cross-section, and it is easily overlooked on the rocky hillsides where it grows. The plant rarely exceeds 25 cm in height, and has clusters of dark red, almost black, flowers at its stem tips. Its foul, carrion-like odour attracts flies, which pollinate it. The seeds are contained in 5 cm long narrow pods. Caralluma is well-known to the hill folk of Oman, who pound up the stems and prepare a tea which is reported to be good for liver ailments. In northern Oman, freshly cut stems of a related species, *Caralluma aucheriana*, are placed on burns to ease pain. In other parts of the country, its juice is used to curdle fresh milk, which is given to the sick for convalescence and as a general tonic. *C. retrospeciens*, a related species with purple flowers and carrion scent, is found northwest of Taif and in north-western Saudi Arabia.

CLEOME

Cleome arabica
Arabic: *'efeina*

A herb with reddish flower heads, found in Saudi Arabia. Cooked in water and applied to a wound, the plant is said to prevent inflammation. According to Musil, it grows on slopes in the valley of al-Washshashe, in hollows south of al-Bishri, and sparsely in a stony district northwest of the peak of al-Zbeit.

COLOCYNTH

Citrullus colocynthis

Arabic: Plant: *shary* (Eastern Arabia), *shuri* (Oman), *hanzal* (elsewhere in the Middle East);
   fruit: *hedeg* (Oman)

Other English: Wild Watermelon

This member of the Gourd family is a curbit of the same genus as the watermelon. The fruit are round white or yellow gourds resembling tennis-balls. Poisonous if taken in quantity, it is extremely bitter and the main source of the purgative colocynth, now no longer favoured because of its potency, but still exported from North Africa, and still carried in the pharmacopoeia.

Colocynths are found growing in northern Arabia, in the desert between al-Jawf and Tayma'. The Bedouins, perhaps tongue in cheek, say this drastic cathartic is so powerful that it is sufficient to cut one of the gourds in half and trample on it to achieve the desired effect. It is also reportedly used as an insecticide. Doughty reported: 'In the better dieted Arabian towns ... these Aarab purge themselves with seeds of the colocynth, but it is only when they have great need, and few times in their lives: the pulp is very bitterness.

Suppositories made of it are said to be effectual for sick languishing of robust persons.' In central Arabia, the roots are mashed with some of the pulp and mixed with goat's milk, and then used as a purge to treat colic. In the United Arab Emirates, the colocynth's seeds are acclaimed as a cure for diabetes.

In Oman, a small amount of the juice is taken as a drastic purge. In the northern part of that country, fresh leaves are placed on the site of scorpion stings and insect bites to relieve pain and itching. Also, the seeds are crushed and made into a poultice to treat tumours and fistulae after they have been cauterized.

In Yemen, the plant is diluted with other ingredients for use as a purge. Its dried, crushed pulp is also blended with oil and used as a salve for joint pain. Early Muslim sources report that the plant was used to treat elephantiasis and other ailments.

CORN POPPY

Papaver dubium or *P. rhoeas*

Arabic: *shaqa'iq al-nu'man*

This central Arabian plant, relative of the opium poppy, is poisonous to livestock but the seeds are sometimes used as a tonic for horses and infusions from the fruits are said to be good for coughs. It can also be used as an eye lotion for animals. Red ink is obtained from the petals.

DESERT BUGLOSS

Echidum horridum
Arabic: *kahal, kahil, kahla'*

A member of the Forget-Me-Not or Borage family, this medicinal plant, found in central Saudi Arabia, is said to relieve urinary complaints and fever. This plant shares its Arabic name with *Arnebia* *decumbens*, because of its similarly red-staining root. Red dye is obtainable from the surface of the taproot of both plants. Bedouin girls sometimes rub the fresh root on their faces, as rouge.

DOGBANE

Rhazya stricta
Arabic: *harmal, hamf, hamd*

A member of this family grows in eastern and central Saudi Arabia and in eastern Yemen (Harib area). A traditional medicinal herb, it was once considered effective in treating venereal diseases. The dried leaves were smoked in a pipe, sometimes mixed with other kinds of leaves, to cure syphilis.

Today, some Bedouin elders still smoke the herb in a pipe, but as a reliable treatment for rheumatism. The plant is considered somewhat toxic. Livestock avoid it. But it is not regarded as a serious threat.

In Najd, the plant has dark green foliage and can give the desert an almost lush look even in summer. In the United Arab Emirates, the herb is used in small quantities to relieve upset stomachs. (*See* Harmel)

DWARF MALLOW

Malva neglecta
Arabic: *khubbayz*

An annual plant of European origin that grows as a weed along roadsides and on waste ground in Oman and elsewhere in the Gulf region. This species is said to contain tannin and is used in folk medicine as a purgative and anti-inflammatory. It is known as *khubbayz*, 'little baker', in some Arabian Gulf countries because its disc-like fruits resemble flat Arabic bread loaves.

GUM ARABIC see ACACIA

HARMEL

Peganum harmala

Arabic: *harmal, khiyyays* ('stinkweed', among the Sulaib), *shajarat al-khunayzir* ('piglet bush', in the North), *chabeeza* or *chah'ess* (Central Arabia)

Other English: Wild Rue, Syrian Rue, Mountain Rue

The plant grows in Arabia, Syria, North Africa, Iran and southern Europe. Today it is well known in central and northern Arabia and Iraq but rare in the eastern part of the Arabian Peninsula. It is found in Kuwait, but only rarely. Harmel has a long history of uses in traditional Arabian medicine. Said to be more tender than ordinary rue and extremely bitter to the taste, the plant contains toxic alkaloids, but is not regarded as a serious problem for livestock. Harmel seed was used by al-Batriq to remove moisture and heat from the body. Al-Kindi used the leaves, seeds and juice in various prescriptions, including remedies for insanity and epilepsy, baldness and haemorrhoids. Harmel seeds are today used as an alterative and purifying medicine, and as an aphrodisiac. The seeds are also regarded as an emmenagogue, diuretic and vomitive.

HELIOTROPE

Heliotropium ramosissimum

Arabic: *ram-ram*

Other English: Turnsole

A member of the Forget-Me-Not or Borage family, this plant is a medicinal in eastern and central Saudi Arabia. In the Eastern Province, it has been used as a remedy for snake bite. In earlier times, snake-bite victims would be given heliotrope tea while a poultice of the plant's leaves was applied to the bite. According to traditional lore, the desert monitor lizard (*Varanus*) acquired immunity from poisonous snakes by eating the plant's leaves and rolling in its branches. But according to Mandaville, medical evidence is lacking, and the treatment probably only has psychological value. Victims of the small common sand viper (*Cerastes cerastes*) usually recover without treatment. Dickson also reports that heliotrope is used as an infusion or paste to treat mouth sores. This practice continues today in central Saudi Arabia, where the plant is boiled in water and used as a mouthwash to cure sore gums and mouth blisters. Similar uses for *H. bacciferum*.

JERICHO ROSE

Anastatica hierochuntica

Arabic: *kaffah, kaff maryam* ('Mary's hand'), *birkan, barukan* (Shammar tribe), *jumay' fatimah* ('Fatimah's fist', Rwala tribe), *kaff al-'adhra'* ('Virgin's hand'), *kafn, qufay'ah* ('Shriveled one', Qahtani tribe), *qunayfidhah* ('Little hedgehog', northern Arabia)

This plant is rather inconspicuous when green, but in the dry season it takes on a characteristic woody, globe form that makes it easy to recognize. It resembles a clutched human hand, and in Arabian folklore is likened to the hand of the Virgin Mary during childbirth; the folk tales say Mary clutched the plant while giving birth.

The dried plant's branches expand and straighten when soaked in water. Jericho rose is used as a herbal remedy in the Arabian Peninsula, and its tea is said to ease childbirth. It is also used as a good-luck charm for the same purpose. Mandaville reports it is sold dried in jars in herbalists' shops of Saudi Arabia's Eastern Province.

LEMON GRASS

Cymbopogon commutatus

Arabic: *sakhbar* (among the 'Utaybah and al-Dawasir tribes), *idhkhir* (among al-Dawasir; also historical), *khasab* (Qahtani tribe) and *hamra'* (Rwala tribe)

A perennial aromatic grass with a history of medicinal use in Arabia. It is probably used most commonly today in an infusion or tea. Mandaville finds no record of lemon grass oil extraction in north-eastern Arabia, though he reports seeing small bunches of the grass sold in a herbalist shop in Dammam. Al-Kindi used lemon grass in a kidney remedy. Some Arabs use lemon grass in cataplasms for stomach tumours. The root, mixed with oxymel syrup, is said to be good for fevers.

MILKWEED

Periploca aphylla

Arabic: *sowas*

One species of the Milkweed family is regarded as medicinal in central Saudi Arabia, and is said to have cardiotonic properties.

MYRTLE
Myrtus communis
Arabic: *as, yas* (Oman)

An aromatic Mediterranean shrub introduced to the Arabian Peninsula. A dense evergreen that grows up to three metres high, it has white flowers and round, blue-black berries. The leaves contain a bitter, aromatic oil that is distilled as an essence in some countries. Villagers in Oman collect the leaves, dry them and beat them to a powder used for its aromatic properties. It is also known to have medicinal properties, and is still found in the pharmacopeias. Avicenna recommended myrtle as an astringent. Its traditional Middle Eastern medicinal uses include as an internal stimulant, antispasmodic and diaphoretic, and as an external rubifacient.

RAT-TAIL PLANTAIN
Plantago major
Arabic: *barhanj, lisan al-kalb*
Other English: Greater Plantain, Common Plantain

The leaves and seeds are used medicinally. The leaves contain tannins and iridoid glycosides, particularly aucubin, which induces uric acid secretion from the kidneys. The seeds contain mucilage, which works as a laxative, and are used to remedy dysentery and diarrhoea.

Known to grow in the al-Hasa area. The seeds are used in Iraq for making poultices to treat boils.

SAFFLOWER
Carthamus oxyacantha
Arabic: *jau'zahr, 'usfur*

Several species of this genus are known as medicinal plants in central, eastern and southern Arabia. *Carthamus oxyacantha* is called in Arabic *jau'zahr* and *'usfur* ('yellow-tint'). This latter name is also applied to *C. tinctorius*, a dye plant widely cultivated in southern Arabia. *C. tinctorius* is known among the Shammar tribe as *samnah* ('butterweed').

Al-Kindi used safflower as part of a salve for wounds incurred by beating with a lash.

SENNA

Cassia italica
Arabic: *ishriq*
Other English: Mecca Senna

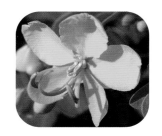

A plant of Arabian origin, whose yellow-green leaves smell tea-like but have no marked taste. As an infusion, they are said to induce nausea and make a useful mild purgative. The plant is widely acknowledged in Bahrain as medicinal. Its pods and leaves are used there as a purgative, and can be purchased in Bahrain's Suq Hawaj. Senna is apparently not used as a medicine today in the nearby Eastern Province of Saudi Arabia, where some Bedouins regard it as toxic to livestock. However, in the past, some in the Eastern Province made it a habit to drink senna liquid (boiled from the leaves) once a month to cleanse the digestive system. In central Saudi Arabia, the seeds of the senna plant are eaten by Bedouins who say they are good for the stomach. The plant also grows on Saudi Arabia's southwestern coastal plain, the Tihama, where it is known for the laxative yielded by its leaves and pods. The seeds are used as a laxative in the United Arab Emirates; Bedouins there claim it cures stomach pains of all kinds. In his day, Avicenna prescribed senna as a purgative for expelling black bile. In modern times, the leaves are exported from Egypt to Europe, where they are used as the drug 'dog senna'.

SIMPLE-LEAVED BEAN CAPER

Zygophyllum simplex
Arabic: *harm, um thirib, hamd, qarmal*

A member of the Caltrops family, the plant is medicinal and possibly good for diabetes. Many grow in Wadi Hair, 60 km south of Riyadh. Its Arabic name *harm* is also used for *Zygophyllum qatarense* and *Z. mandavillei*.

SMOOTH SOW-THISTLE

Sonchus oleraceus
Arabic: *adheed* (Bahrain), *khuwwaysh* (eastern Saudi Arabia)

Found in eastern Saudi Arabia and Bahrain. Related to the common dandelion, this plant contains a milky sap which is believed to possess magical properties. The leaves are edible, and in Bahrain are cooked or eaten raw in salads.

SODOM APPLE *see* APPLE OF SODOM

SPURGE

Euphorbia helioscopia and *E. resinifera*, among others
Arabic: *furbiyun, afarbiyun*
Other English: Euphorbium

Euphorbium, a classical name from Euphorbus, physician to Juba, king of Mauritania. A common weed in West Asia. Its juice is poisonous, so its use in traditional medicine is rare. Al-Kindi used euphorbium resin in ointment for abscesses, fistulas and scrofula, and in a remedy for insanity. Al-Bitriq used ephorbium to remove phlegm, moistness and heat from the body. Al-Razi, however, regarded euphorbium as a poison to be watched. Avicenna mentions *Euphorbia pityusa*, grown in Morocco, a cactus-like plant that produces an acid resin which was used medicinally as an emetic and purgative, to expel 'yellow water'. In Egypt today, spurge is used only externally as a rubbing agent to counteract paralysis and apoplexy.

TAMARISK

Tamarix arabica
Arabic: Tree: *al-tarfa'*; gall: *thamar al-tarfa', harmarij, jazmazaj, 'adhbah*

All parts of the tamarisk tree were widely used in ancient Babylonian medicine. Al-Kindi used tamarisk gall (gallnut) in a tooth powder for polishing the teeth, for removing the decayed parts of teeth, for halitosis and general protection of the mouth. Today, tamarisk gall is used in the Middle East for haemorrhage, dysentery, the eyes and in dentifrices.

WITHANIA

Withania somnifera
Arabic: *haml balbul, shaukaran*
Other English: Winter Cherry

The roots are used medicinally. A sedative narcotic, whose principal active alkaloid is somniferine. While little known in the West, it has a wide variety of medicinal uses in India, holding an important place in Ayurvedic medicine. Mandaville says: 'It is not, apparently, highly toxic but should be treated with some respect.' Levey identifies it with henbane, and notes that it is used for scorpion stings, toothache, swelling, stomach ailments, strangury, and as a tonic and an aphrodisiac. It is particularly noted for its intoxicating properties. Al-Hasa gardeners call the fruit *bulbul*, according to Mandaville.

NATURAL BEAUTY

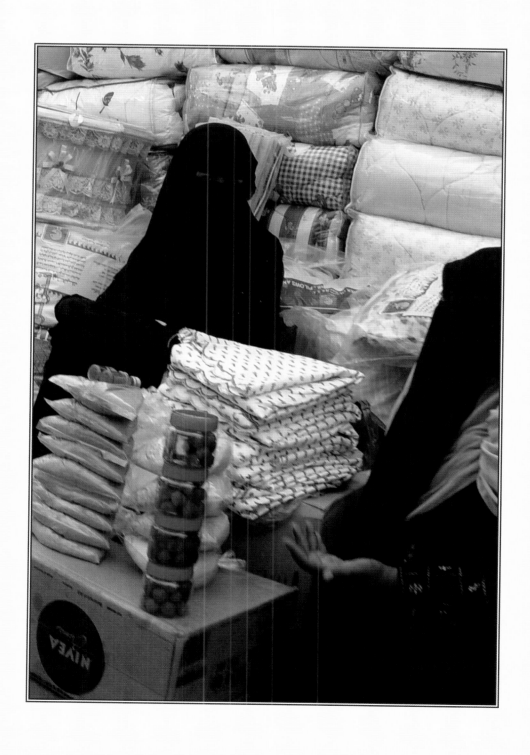

HAIR CARE

Aloe

🌢 *Aloe vera* gel mixed with *sidr* and pomegranate peelings makes for beautiful healthy hair. (KSA)

Arugula *(jarjeer)*

🌢 Used in salads it is good for the blood, skin, and hair. The oil nourishes and strengthens the hair. (Bahrain)

🌢 Blend with water to strengthen the hair. (Western KSA)

🌢 To strengthen hair, massage arugula oil into the scalp. (Central KSA)

🌢 Arugula oil thickens the hair. As a vegetable, it contains vitamins and is rich in iron. (Central KSA)

🌢 *Jarjeer* juice strengthens hair. It is rubbed or massaged into the scalp. (Northern KSA)

Basil

🌢 For a pleasant odour in hair, clothes, and house, use *mashmum*. (KSA)

🌢 Older women used to put basil under their hair to give it a nice smell. (Southern KSA)

🌢 For hair care, 'my mother used henna and a mixture of roses, basil and *al-ful*, a small white flower called Arabian jasmine [*Jasminum sambac*], and she mixed it and put it on her hair.' (Central KSA)

Black Seed

🌢 Black seed oil nourishes the hair and it helps it grow. (Western KSA)

🌢 I don't use black seed, but I use black seed oil. I apply it on my eyelashes and eyebrows every night before bed. It helps nourish the hair and helps it grow. (Western KSA)

🌢 For healthy hair, use black seed in a mixture of shampoo, honey and yoghurt. (Southern KSA)

🌢 Use black seed with sesame oil. Apply black seed oil to your hair. (Western KSA)

Chamomile

🌢 To strengthen and stimulate the growth of hair and make it shiny and silky, boil chamomile with water and add nettle. Leave it boiling then mix it with powdered henna. Leave it until it becomes warm, apply to the hair and leave for 4-6 hours. Wash the hair well then rub hair and scalp with olive oil. Wash with shampoo. (Eastern KSA)

Garlic

᠊᠊ After shampooing, use vinegar with water in the final rinse for shiny and healthy hair. Add to the mixture onion, vanilla and lemon to clean and treat the scalp. Grind garlic in a mixture of oils (olive, cucumber). Leave it under the sun in a covered bottle for one day, then apply to hair and cover for one hour before washing. The bad smell will last for about a week. (Western KSA)

Hibiscus

᠊᠊ Mix henna with hibiscus (boiled in water). Mix and put in hair. This makes a red colour. (Northern KSA)

᠊᠊ Boil hibiscus then take its water and mix it with henna for colouring hair a brown to red colour. (Central KSA)

᠊᠊ Henna leaves are ground and mixed with water or hibiscus or tea or lemon and put on hair for four hours. (Eastern KSA)

Mahaleb Cherry

᠊᠊ For beautiful, healthy hair, use oils, henna and mahaleb *(Prunus mahaleb)*. (Eastern KSA)

᠊᠊ My grandmother used roses, after grinding them as a cream, to soften the hair. Also mahaleb and nutmeg are used for the same purpose. After grinding and mixing them with water, put them in the hair as a cream. (Eastern KSA)

Rose

᠊᠊ Use dried fruits of the rose *(mishat)*. (Central KSA)

᠊᠊ Mother used henna and a mixture of roses, basil and *al-ful* [a small white flower called Arabian jasmine, *Jasminum sambac*], and she mixed it and put it on her hair. (Central KSA)

᠊᠊ Grandmother used henna and meat fat by rubbing them on the hair, then washing. Also, she used a special mixture of a tablespoon of parsley juice, a tablespoon of onion juice, and sesame oil, and rubbed the head with it and exposed it to the sun to kill lice and eggs. Also, she used rose after grinding it as a cream to soften the hair. Also mahaleb and nutmeg are used for the same purpose, after grinding and mixing them with water, then putting in the hair as a cream. (Eastern KSA)

Sidr

᠊᠊ For beautiful hair, our mothers used *sidr*, aloe vera and pomegranate peelings. (Southern KSA)

᠊᠊ Use *sidr* to wash the hair and make it smooth and silky. (Eastern KSA)

HENNA

Across Arabia, henna is used in a great variety of ways as an aid to health and beauty – as a cosmetic, for decoration, to nourish and strengthen hair, or as a hair dye.

Hair Care and Colouring

- Use henna, black seeds, *sidr*, oil, honey and eggs to nourish and strengthen the hair. (Bahrain)
- My grandmother used *sidr* water and henna water. (Northern KSA)
- I use henna for the hair by drying the leaves and grinding them to powder, mixing them with water and oil and putting it on the hair. (Southern KSA)
- Black seed is used with henna for the hair. (Southern KSA)
- Henna stimulates hair growth and thickness. This is how to do it: mix henna with warm water. Let it stand, then put it on the hair and leave it for 6-7 hours. (Southern KSA)
- To make your hair stronger and help prevent hair loss, you mix henna with water and put it over all your hair and leave it for 4 hours. Then clean it. Do this once a month. (Central KSA)
- I use henna because it gives the hair a natural colour and a good fragrance. Also, it strengthens the hair and prevents hair loss. And I apply some oils to the hair. (Central KSA)
- *Sidr* and henna are moistened with warm water and left for half an hour. After that, both are used to wash the hair. Henna is used for the hands too. (Eastern KSA)
- My mother and grandmother used henna plants. They used this plant as a hair colouring to cover white hairs and make hair stronger and healthier. They would cut 3-4 black lemons into small parts then boil them twice and mix them with henna. Leave the mixture for some time. (Eastern KSA)
- We use henna to treat many conditions. One is headache: put henna on head. For hair colouring: also put henna on head. It works to remove impurities from the scalp, like microbes, parasites and dandruff. (Eastern KSA)
- Use henna to treat headache and dandruff and to strengthen the hair and colour it. The leaves are ground and mixed with water or hibiscus or tea or lemon and put on hair for four hours. (Eastern KSA)
- My grandmother used henna and meat fat by rubbing them in the hair and then washing. Also, she used a special mixture of a tablespoon of parsley juice,

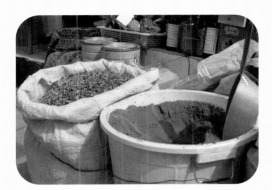

a tablespoon of onion juice, and sesame oil, and rubbed the head with it and exposed it to the sun to kill lice and their eggs. Also, she used rose, grinding it into a cream to soften the hair. (Eastern KSA)

- Henna is used to colour and nourish the hair. It's also used for cracks in the hands and feet. (Southern KSA)
- Henna is to colour the white hair and give it a healthy look. I don't like the red color of henna so I make my own mixture. I mix henna with black coffee, Turkish coffee, boiled tea and leave the mixture covered for one night, then put it on my hair for 2-3 hours. (Western KSA)
- I put henna on my hair twice a month. I keep the henna on my hair for four hours, then wash my hair with water only. After that, I apply either olive oil or sesame oil on my hair and leave it overnight. This keeps my hair from losing its natural oils and enhances the deep red colour of the henna. (Western KSA)
- Use henna to beautify hair. (Northern KSA)

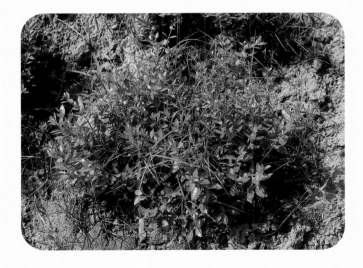

HENNA

Decoration

🍂 Henna is used to colour and feed the hair. It's also used to treat cracks in hands and feet. (Southern KSA)

🍂 Henna is used to decorate hands, and is prepared by mixing henna with dried sidr with a little water until it becomes soft. You can add a few drops of lemon juice. Adding lemon makes the colour stronger. Henna is very useful for the hair as well. (Central KSA)

🍂 I use henna to colour the hands. This is what makes women more special than men. As Prophet Muhammad said, by drying the leaves and grinding them and mixing them with water. Then put it on the hands for two hours or more. (Southern KSA)

🍂 Henna is used to decorate hands and is prepared by mixing henna with dried sidr with a small amount of water until it becomes soft. You can add a few drops of lemon juice. Adding lemon will help to make the colour stronger. Henna is very useful for the hair. (Central KSA)

🍂 We use henna the conventional way by adding eggs, oil and other ingredients. If I want to colour my hair, I do not add the other ingredients. If I want to nourish or moisturize and not colour my hair, I oil my hair continuously to restore vitality and body, especially when it is dry. (Bahrain)

🍂 Henna is used to decorate hands and feet. This is how to prepare it: Grind dried henna leaves into powder or buy ready-made powder. Mix a full glass of water with a full glass of henna until the henna becomes soft. Then use it immediately. (Southern KSA)

🍂 Use henna for decorating. Mixing a quantity of henna with water until you have a firm dough. Decorate hands and feet or colour the hair. For hair colouring, mix henna with a lot of water until it becomes liquid and put it in the hair. (Southern KSA)

MAHALEB PERFUME

❧ Clean, grind and sieve mahaleb and *wurss* (a fragrant wood). Mix $^1/_2$ cup mahaleb, $^1/_2$ cup *wurss*, $^1/_4$ seed nutmeg, and some saffron in a mortar. Pound until ingredients blend together. Place a live coal and a piece of snail inside the mortar in order to smoke the blend. Tightly cover the mortar to hold the smoke inside. Leave for 1 or 2 hours. Pour mixture into a container, cover it, and keep it in a dry, dark place until needed. To use, mix a small amount with some rose water and apply on forehead. (Oman)

❧ Mix and grind together mahaleb, basil, small roses, cloves and cardamom. Mix with water and apply to skin. (Southern KSA)

COSMETICS

❧ Use castor oil to thicken the eye lashes, twice a week. (Western KSA)

❧ Mother used turmeric and that was her makeup and musk (perfume), basil, roses – all that was her perfume and kohl was ground as powder and put in a kohl container and she put kohl around the eyes and she also massaged her body with olive oil. (Central KSA)

❧ My mother put saffron on her lips and cheeks. (Central KSA)

❧ I apply turmeric on my eyelashes and eyebrows every night before bed. (KSA)

❧ I apply black seed oil on my eyelashes and eyebrows every night before bed. It helps nourish the hair and makes it grow. (Western KSA)

❧ Put drops of rose water on a cucumber slice and apply to the eyes for rejuvenation. (Eastern KSA)

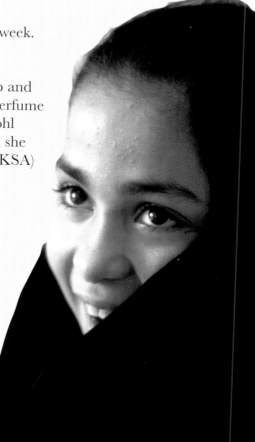

SKIN CARE

Arugula (*jarjeer*)

🐾 I use natural oils such as *jarjeer* oil and coconut oil, and I use henna once a month. (Eastern KSA)

Chickpea

🐾 Mix chickpea flour with rose water. Apply to skin and leave on until it dries. Rinse with warm water. This tightens pores and leaves skin clean, soft and beautiful. (Eastern KSA)

Cucumber

🐾 For beautiful skin, I use cucumber, jarjeer and yoghurt. (Western KSA)
🐾 For healthy skin, I use honey, yoghurt, cucumber and fenugreek. My mother also used fenugreek. (Southern KSA)
🐾 For oily skin, use lemon as a cleanser; cucumbers as an astringent. For dry skin, use milk as a cleanser, sweet almond oil as a moisturizer. (Bahrain)
🐾 For beautiful, healthy skin, mix cucumber and yoghurt and use it as a mask. (Southern KSA)
🐾 Mix honey, yoghurt, cucumber and fenugreek for healthy skin. (Southern KSA)
🐾 For healthy skin, use cucumber, *jarjeer* (arugula) and yoghurt. (Western KSA)

Black seed

🐾 My mother used a mixture of ground black seed and honey as a paste. Apply it on the face and expose it to the sun for a short time during the day. Then wash. (Eastern KSA)
🐾 Mix a little powdered black seed with a little natural olive oil. Then, cover the face and neck and expose to cool sun rays for 20 minutes. Then, wash it off. This keeps your skin beautiful. (Southern KSA)

Cumin

🐾 Washing one's face with a solution of cumin beautifies the skin. (Eastern KSA)

Honey

🐾 I use a mask of honey for 15 minutes, then wash it with warm water and dry it. Then I rub my face with a little olive oil. Also, I use a mask containing yoghurt, yeast and vinegar by putting it on the face and neck until it dries, then washing with warm water and putting some drops of rose water and slices of cucumber on the eyes. I make natural exfoliant for my face with oat, drops of lemon juice, grated apple and some yoghurt. Then, I massage my face very well, then I add some drops of water and complete the massage to stimulate blood circulation, then wash. (Eastern KSA)
🐾 Use honey, sidr and lemon to clean the skin. (Southern KSA)
🐾 To clean the skin, use honey, lemon and mahaleb (*Prunus mahaleb* or perfumed cherry). (Northern KSA)

🌰 Use honey, olive oil and lemon, in addition to creams. (Southern KSA)

🌰 For beautiful, healthy skin, use honey, yoghurt, cucumber, fenugreek. (Southern KSA)

🌰 For healthy skin, use yeast, yoghurt and honey. Mix one spoon of yeast with hot water then add one spoon of yoghurt and one spoon of honey. Apply to the face. Leave on until it dries, then scrub your face with your hand and wash. (Western KSA)

🌰 I use olive oil because it's helpful and nourishing for the skin. Also, I use honey and drops of orange juice for a mask. (Northern KSA)

🌰 I beat eggs and use as a mask. I mix honey with yoghurt and also use as a mask. (Western KSA)

🌰 Use honey, rose water, olive oil and almond oil for healthy skin. (Western KSA)

🌰 I eat healthy food rich in vitamins, proteins, carbohydrates, etc. Each week I apply a mask of honey for 15 minutes then wash my face with warm water and dry it. Then I rub my face with a little olive oil. Also, I use a mask containing yoghurt, yeast and vinegar. I put it on my face and neck until it dries, then I wash with warm water and put some drops of rose water and slices of cucumber on the eyes. (Eastern KSA)

Myrrh

🌰 Use myrrh and honey. (Central KSA)

🌰 Myrrh is for stomach pain and healthy skin especially. (Northern KSA)

Saffron

🌰 My grandmother used saffron with safflowers. She mixed them with water. She put them on her face like a mask. (Central KSA)

Turmeric

🌰 In the past, they used mud and stones for cleaning. Then, they washed their bodies and put on some turmeric (yellow) and washed the hair with powdered dried sidr. (Central KSA)

🌰 In the past, people cleaned their bodies naturally with sidr, lemon, turmeric with olive oil and henna. (Northern KSA)

🌰 Mix a quantity of turmeric with a little water until you have a soft dough. Then, put it on the face for 10-15 minutes. Remove it with water. It prevents the skin from becoming dark. (Southern KSA)

🌰 For beautiful healthy skin, use turmeric and butter. (Northern KSA)

🌰 Put honey on your face and massage it. Steam your face with olive oil rubbed on the face. Turmeric with milk will whiten the skin. (Eastern KSA)

Rose

🌰 Use rose water and olive oil. (Central KSA) Use honey, rose water, olive oil, almond oil. (Western KSA)

🌰 Mother used yoghurt, honey, rose water with starch (cornflour). (Central KSA)

🌰 Grandmother used boiled leaves and flowers of the rose for her skin beauty. (Eastern KSA)

🌰 Clean the skin and face with rose water or flower water. (Central KSA)

RECIPES

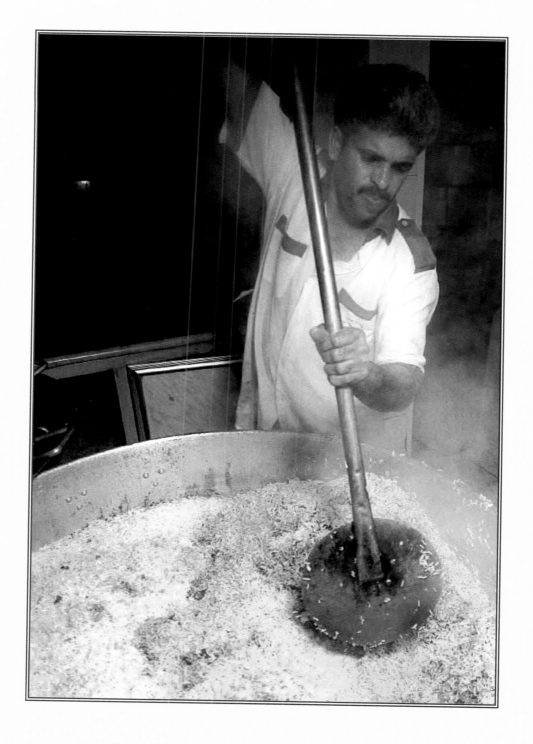

Rice is prepared for a wedding party.

BEVERAGES

Arabic Coffee
(Hail, Northern Province)

1 tablespoon coffee for each cup of water
Saffron threads

1 tablespoon cardamom for each 1 $^1/_2$ cups water

Roast coffee beans to a light brown color. Crush them to a coarse grain. Coarsely grind cardamom. Put roasted, ground coffee beans into cold water. Bring to a boil. Boil for 5 to 7 minutes and allow to settle. Pour into a serving pot and add cardamom plus a sprinkle (4 to 6 threads) of saffron. Bring to a slight boil again and serve.

🐜 🐜 🐜 🐜

Arabic Coffee
Hanan Anbur (Dammam, Eastern Province)

In a cooking dallah *(coffee pot):*

water to boil
1 teaspoon cardamom

3 tablespoons coffee powder
$^1/_2$ teaspoon saffron

In a serving dallah:

1 teaspoon cardamom
$^1/_2$ teaspoon saffron

Fill a serving dallah with water to measure the amount. Then, pour the water into a cooking dallah. Add an extra $^1/_2$ cup of water because some will evaporate. Bring to a rapid boil and add 3 tablespoons coffee powder. (If using a dark coffee powder, never add more than 3 tablespoons). Add a teaspoon of cardamom with a $^1/_2$ teaspoon of saffron. Leave to boil 20-30 minutes.

Meanwhile, add a teaspoon of cardamom and $^1/_2$ teaspoon saffron to a serving dallah or thermos. Turn off the fire. Let sit 1-2 minutes so the coffee falls to the bottom. Pour into a service dallah.

Note: You may also add $^1/_8$ teaspoon of clove powder with coffee, if desired.

🐜 🐜 🐜 🐜

Arabic Coffee with Nakhwa

Fatin Hareth (Najran, Southern Province)

'Nakhwah (ajwain) is usually added to Arabic coffee.'

5 cups boiled water   3 tablespoons Arabic coffee
1 teaspoon dried, powdered ginger   2 teaspoons cardamom
Saffron   Nakhwa

Boil ginger and coffee in water for 10-15 minutes.   In the thermos, put 2 teaspoons of cardamom and some saffron and also *nakhwa (ajwain)*. Pour coffee into the thermos and prepare to serve.

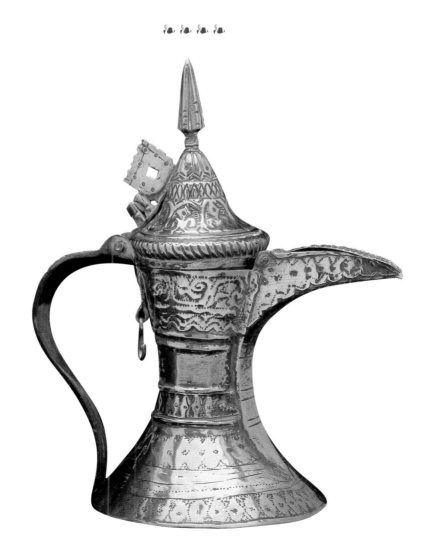

Arabic Coffee
Khadija Al-Balkhy (Western Province)

Boil six cups of water. Add three tablespoons of freshly-ground roasted coffee beans. Allow the mixture to boil up to the rim a couple of times or until its aroma fills the place. Remove from the heat. Put half a tablespoon of ground cardamom into a brass or silver serving coffee pot and then add the boiled coffee mixture. Allow to settle for a minute before drinking.

Sweet Coffee
Najah Sendi (Makkah, Western Province)

12 tablespoons powdered milk (Nido or Anchor)
5 tablespoons sugar (add more or less to taste)
4 tablespoons chopped almonds
3 to 4 tablespoons rice flour (add more if you like thicker coffee)
Roasted ground almonds or ground cinnamon to sprinkle on top (optional)

8 cups water
1 teaspoon ground cardamom

Dilute the powdered milk in water. Put in a pan and bring to a boil. Lower the heat to low-medium. Add the rice flour while stirring. Stir until the milk slightly thickens (if the milk doesn't thicken, increase heat to medium-high). As soon as the coffee thickens, stir in the sugar then add almonds and cardamom. Sprinkle with roasted almonds or ground cinnamon. Serve hot and enjoy.

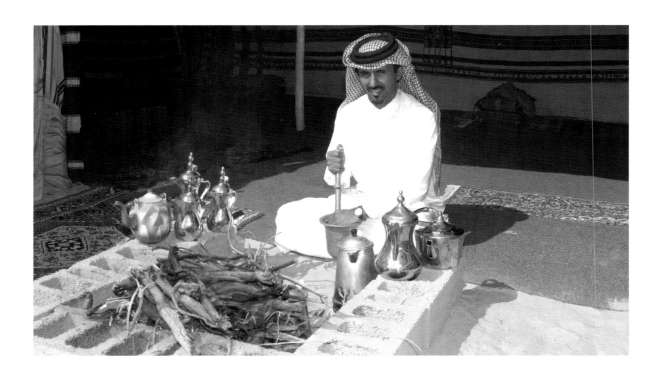

Omani Coffee

Start with 1 kg. coffee beans and 1 cup cardamom. Roast coffee beans until brown. Add cardamom and stir. Finely grind and keep in glass container, or you may grind coffee at the time you wish to make coffee.

Preparation of coffee:
4-6 cups water
3 cups ground coffee
1 coffee cup cardamom powder

Boil water. Add ground roasted coffee beans and boil on low fire until froth disappears. Stir in cardamom. Remove from heat and let stand for a few minutes. Pour into coffee pot or thermos.

Note: Saffron, cardamom or rose water is sometimes added to the coffee pot before pouring coffee into it. In Dhofar, Oman, cloves or ginger are added. In some areas of interior Oman, a small amount of sandal (sandalwood) oil is added.

Lime-Mint Drink
Aisha Kay (al-Khobar, Eastern Province)

6 medium limes
6-8 fresh mint leaves, chopped
5-6 ice cubes

$^3/_4$ to 1 cup sugar
1 litre water

Cut limes in half and squeeze the juice into a sturdy blender container. Add the sugar, chopped mint, water, and ice cubes. Blend at high speed until ice is crushed. Pour mixture into a serving pitcher and add a little more water or sugar to taste.

Ginger Tea with Honey and Lemon
(Saudi Arabia)

Place one tablespoon of fresh grated ginger root with two cups of water in a pan. Cover tightly with lid. Bring to a simmer and gently continue simmering for twenty minutes. Be sure not to boil. Strain and enjoy a lovely, comforting tea.

It is good served plain and absolutely delightful with a tablespoon of honey and the juice of half a lemon added to each cup.

BREAKFAST

Omelette with Banana
Abeer Zaki (Makkah, Western Province)

'This is a very old and traditional recipe from Mecca. I don't think the new generation knows this recipe ... it's very easy ... and very special.'

Put some butter in a pan, then cut the bananas in slices and fry them just a little bit. Then add a couple of eggs and stir. Add a pinch of sugar and salt and a very little amount of cardamom (less than a pinch). Eat this omelette with bread, preferably wheat bread.

❧ ❧ ❧ ❧

Masoub
Kamilia Mandoura (Jeddah, Western Province)

Melt butter in a saucepan. Slice a banana into the pan. Mash when soft, then remove from heat. Cut a slice of wheat bread into very small pieces and mix with the banana. Add sugar as desired. Note: The wheat bread *(khubz burr)* is a thin brown bread with black seed and is widely available in Mecca and Jeddah.

❧ ❧ ❧ ❧

Masoub (Modern Variation)
Kamilia Mandoura (Jeddah, Western Province)

Melt butter in a saucepan. Slice a banana into the pan. Mash when soft, then remove from heat. Add cornflakes and mix. Serve with *gishta* (cream).

SALADS

Cucumber Yoghurt Salad

INGREDIENTS

2 cups yoghurt
2 cloves crushed garlic
paprika

4 cucumbers, peeled and finely diced
salt
1 tablespoon freshly chopped mint

Add diced cucumbers, salt, and crushed garlic cloves to yoghurt. Mix well. Place into serving bowl(s) and chill well. Sprinkle with paprika and garnish with mint before serving.

🐦 🐦 🐦 🐦

Tomato and Cucumber Salad

INGREDIENTS

3 tomatoes
1 onion, chopped
2 tablespoons olive oil
fresh mint
salt

2 cucumbers
$1/4$ cup lemon juice
1 clove garlic
fresh parsley

Mash garlic and salt in a bowl. Add lemon juice, and mix well. Chop onion, tomatoes, and cucumbers into bite-size pieces and add to the garlic mixture. Add chopped mint and parsley along with the olive oil. Mix gently.

🐦 🐦 🐦 🐦

Salatat al-Hummus (Chickpea Salad)
Munira Al-Ashgar (Dhahran, Eastern Province)

INGREDIENTS

1 jar (400g) chickpeas or 1 cup dried chickpeas
3 bundles of parsley, cleaned and chopped
1 green pepper, finely chopped
2 tablespoons white onions, finely chopped

2 green onions, finely chopped
1 cup tomatoes, finely chopped
2 tablespoons mint, finely chopped

Dressing
$1/3$ cup olive oil
2 tablespoons vinegar
salt and pepper to taste

1 teaspoon lemon juice
1 tablespoon sumac

If using dried chickpeas, soak them overnight. Then boil them in salt and water until done. If using chickpeas from the jar, simply drain completely. Mix all ingredients with the chickpeas.

Mix olive oil, lemon juice, vinegar, salt and pepper in a jar and shake well. Mix the dressing with the salad whenever ready to serve.

🐜 🐜 🐜 🐜

Tabbouleh

INGREDIENTS

1 cup burghul (cracked wheat)
2 cups fresh parsley, chopped
1 cup finely chopped spring onions,
    including green parts
$3/4$ cup chopped tomatoes
$1/2$ cup fresh lemon juice

1 cup finely chopped fresh mint
$1/4$ cup finely chopped yellow onions
salt and cayenne pepper
4 cucumbers, finely chopped
$1/2$ cup olive oil

Rinse and dry the burghul, place in a large bowl. Add the chopped tomatoes, cucumbers, onions, parsley and mint. Mix gently. Leave for half an hour to absorb the juices. Add salt and pepper to taste. Add some olive oil and lemon juice, mixing well. Add more lemon, oil, or salt to taste and serve on a platter of lettuce leaves within 15 minutes so that it does not go soggy.

Arugula and Pomegranate Salad
Huda I. Nawwab (Dhahran, Eastern Province)

INGREDIENTS

2 bunches *arugula (jarjeer)*   7 radishes (sliced lengthwise)
1 cup sour pomegranate seeds

Vinaigrette:

3 tablespoons sumac   3 tablespoons olive oil
3 tablespoons vinegar   Dash of salt

Wash arugula and cut off stems. Discard stems and use leaves. Add radish slices and pomegranate seeds. Mix vinaigrette ingredients and keep in a bowl. Set aside for a few hours. Pour vinaigrette over the arugula just before serving. (*The Arabian Sun*, Saudi Aramco, November 20, 2002)

Fattoush

INGREDIENTS

One-half loaf of Arabic flat bread, toasted and broken into pieces
2 large fresh tomatoes, chopped   2 cucumbers, peeled and finely diced
3 spring onions, finely chopped   2 cups purslane, or shredded lettuce leaves
1 tablespoon fresh mint, chopped $1/2$-1 cup parsley, chopped
2 cloves garlic $1/2$ teaspoon cayenne pepper
$1/4$ teaspoon sumac   salt
$1/4$ -$1/2$ cup lemon juice   3 tablespoons olive oil

Mix the chopped tomatoes, cucumbers, onions, purslane, mint, parsley, garlic, cayenne pepper and sumac in a salad bowl. Add salt, olive oil, and lemon juice to taste. Add toasted bits of Arabic bread and mix briskly. Serve while bread is still crisp.

Saudi Cilantro Salad (Serves 2-4)

INGREDIENTS

3 medium tomatoes
$^1/_2$ bunch green coriander leaves (cilantro)
salt to taste

2 green chilli peppers
juice of 2 lemons

Grill tomatoes over low heat. Peel and purée them. Wash coriander and chili peppers. Chop both, then grind using mortar and pestle. Add this mixture to the tomatoes, plus salt and lemon juice. Mix and serve.

❧ ❧ ❧ ❧

Sprouted Fenugreek Seeds

In a glass jar, put 2-3 tablespoons of seeds in 2 cups of water. Cover with muslin or cheesecloth and secure with an elastic band. Soak 8-12 hours. Drain off the water and reserve to drink. Then turn the jar upside down and on an angle to drain. To keep the seeds moist, rinse with water and drain one to two times a day until the seeds sprout. Be sure to roll the jar in your hands each time so the seed is loosened and not sticking together in one mass. When the sprouts are 1-3 cm long (in approximately 2-4 days) they can be eaten as a snack, used as a garnish, or added to tossed salads, potato salads, sandwiches, or stir fries (just before serving). Keep sprouts covered so they do not dry out and lose flavor. Store in refrigerator.

SOUP

Wheat Soup (Shurbat al-Habb)

Nimah Ismail Nawwab (Dhahran, Eastern Province)

INGREDIENTS

$^3/_4$ cup wheat
$1^1/_2$ pounds lamb with bones
5-6 tablespoons tomato paste
2-3 large tomatoes (chopped)
10-12 cups water
1 teaspoon salt
2-3 tablespoons *shaiba* (a blend of dried lichens, easily available in Saudi Arabia - optional)
2 1-inch cinnamon sticks
2-3 cardamom pods
3 cloves
1 teaspoon cumin seeds
6 black peppercorns

Wash the wheat. Put meat, tomato paste, tomatoes and water in a large pot. Bring to a boil. Using a piece of cheesecloth, make a small bundle with the *shaiba* and other spices with the exception of salt. Put the tightly closed bundle in the pot. Cook for 10 minutes over high heat. Reduce heat to minimum and cook for 20-30 minutes. Cover pot and simmer for 2 hours. Add salt and serve with lemon wedges.

🐝 🐝 🐝 🐝

MAIN DISHES

Saliq

Nimah Ismail Nawwab (Dhahran, Eastern Province)

This rice dish is smooth in consistency and is often served with *duqqus* (a hot sauce often made of fresh coriander, hot chili peppers, garlic, tomatoes, and lemon juice) as well as a green salad. Presented to guests at weddings and on special occasions it is served on trays and garnished with liver slices and butter or clarified butter.

INGREDIENTS

liver slices and butter or clarified butter	3 tablespoons oil
3 mastic pellets	2 cardamom pods
12-14 cups boiling water	3 whole chickens (cleaned with skin intact)
dash of lemon salt	5 cups Egyptian rice
1$^1/_2$ chicken bouillon cubes	

1 cup liquid milk (made by mixing 3 tablespoons powdered milk with 1 cup of water)
2 tablespoons butter or $^1/_2$ teaspoon *samn baladi* (clarified butter from lamb)

Heat oil in a large pot. Add mastic pellets and cardamom. After pellets have dissolved, add the whole chickens and pour in boiled water. Keep pot uncovered and cook over high heat for 10 minutes. Spoon off foam as it rises. Cook over medium high for 20 more minutes. Remove chickens from stock and rub them with lemon salt. Keep chickens in an oven platter ready for broiling later on.

Add rice to stock and cook over high heat for 5 minutes. Reduce heat to medium high heat and cook for 20 minutes. Stir rice from time to time especially the rice at the bottom so that it doesn't stick. Start broiling chickens. Broil for 7 minutes, turn over and broil for a further 5 minutes. Continue cooking rice until stock is almost gone. Add the chicken bouillon cube and the milk. Cook for 10 minutes over low heat and keep on warm heat while carving the chicken before serving. The consistency of the rice should resemble that of a smooth rice pudding and the rice is poured onto serving dishes or large deep trays. Top with chicken pieces and clarified or regular butter. Serve with *duqqus* sauce (*see page 191*) as well as a green salad. Serves 10-12 persons. (*The Arabian Sun*, Saudi Aramco, November 20, 2002).

Ghozi (Stuffed Lamb)

Munira Al-Ashgar (Dhahran, Eastern Province)

INGREDIENTS

1 whole young lamb
$^2/_3$ cup almonds
bazaar (mixed spices)
1 cup oil for frying nuts
6 eggs, hard boiled and shelled

2 cups rice
1 whole chicken, boneless and skinned
lemon, salt and curry for cleaning
2 $^1/_3$ cups pine nuts

2 tablespoons bazaar
$^1/_4$ cup rose water
3 teaspoons curry

1 teaspoon saffron
3 teaspoons cardamom
salt and pepper to taste

Clean the lamb repeatedly inside and outside with water. Rub it with salt, lemon and curry. Leave the lamb for one hour. After one hour wash the lamb thoroughly again.

Boil the rice in water and salt until half-done. Strain the rice.

Fry the almonds in the oil. Remove the almonds from the oil and fry the pine nuts in the same oil. Fry the chicken in a small amount of oil. Cut the chicken into cubes.

Mix the rice, nuts, whole eggs and chicken cubes.

Rub the inside of the lamb with mixed spices (bazaar spices).

Stuff $^2/_3$ of the inside of the lamb with the rice mixture. Stitch the lamb closed with large needle and thread. Rub the outside of the lamb with spices, saffron and salt.

Wrap the lamb in heavy aluminum foil many times and place in a tray two inches deep.

Place in a preheated oven set at 500°F. (260°C.) for one hour. Reduce the heat to 400°F. (204°C.) and leave for two hours. Finally reduce the heat to 350°F. (177°C.) and allow to cook for three hours.

Place parsley leaves on a tray and place the cooked lamb over the parsley and garnish with green pepper, boiled eggs and tomatoes.

[*Note*: To determine the age of the lamb inspect the teeth. The teeth of the lamb must be small in size.]

Chicken Kabsa (Serves 4-6)
(Eastern Province)

INGREDIENTS

1 whole chicken
2 cups Basmati rice
3 onions
1-3 tablespoons tomato paste
2 tomatoes, chopped
dried limes (loomi)
spring onions
2 green chili peppers
cooking oil
1/2 teaspoon cumin
coriander seeds
bazaar spice (special mix available in Mid-Eastern supermarkets)

small piece ginger root
coriander seeds
3-4 cardamom seed pods
1/2 teaspoon red pepper
cinnamon sticks
8-10 black peppercorns
3 bay leaves
1/8 teaspoon turmeric
6-8 whole cloves
salt to taste
1 small can (8 oz.) tomato paste

Onion Topping:

1/2 tablespoon butter
3 spring onions

1 medium chopped onion
sultanas, pine nuts, almonds

Rinse and soak Basmati rice. It can be soaked in advance for thirty minutes or for several hours.

Sprinkle bazaar spice on chicken and place in a large pot with one finely chopped onion, a small piece of chopped ginger root, 3-4 cardamom seed pods, a sprinkle of coriander seeds, and 1/2 teaspoon red pepper. Start browning meat on stove. Add 3 small 1/2 size sticks of cinnamon and 8-10 black peppercorns (as desired). Add 3 bay leaves, 1/8 teaspoon or less of turmeric, 6-8 whole cloves, and 1/2 teaspoon cumin.

Meanwhile, in another small pan, fry the second onion in 2 tablespoons cooking oil. When translucent, remove oil. Add chopped tomatoes and sprinkle with salt. While still cooking, add 1/2 cup tomato paste. Carefully puncture one side of 2-3 black lemons. Combine all ingredients and put mixture into the chicken pot. Add another 1/2 cup tomato paste and about 4 cups hot water. Cover.

Cook rice with 1 tablespoon salt and 1 tablespoon oil. Add two 2-inch long cinnamon sticks and 1 cardamom pod. Boil for 7-10 minutes. Drain into rice sieve. Cover with plate to let steam. After 10 minutes, add rice to meat mixture.

Add more water to the chicken mixture, if needed. Add a coarsely chopped onion. Top with 2 green chilies. Water is being absorbed at this point. Heat is at medium high.

When ready, remove hot peppers and onions from dish. Place rice on serving dish. Then, put chicken on top of the rice to serve. Garnish with pine nut, sultana, almond and onion topping.

Onion Topping:

Add $^1/_2$ tablespoon butter to small pan with 1 medium chopped onion. Cook onion. Add handful (as desired) of sultanas. Add 3 spring onions, coarsely chopped. Add 4 tablespoons pine nuts and three tablespoons almonds (previously soaked to remove salt and then peeled and chopped).

Cheese Pie
Claudine Shane (USA/Lebanon)

INGREDIENTS

1 package puff pastry
haloumi cheese, grated
1 egg
parsley or mint (optional)

mozzarella cheese, grated
$^3/_4$ cup milk
black seed

Divide a package of puff pastry into two. Layer a pie tin with half of the puff pastry. Pour the grated cheese (one package each, or amount desired) into the pie tin. Add freshly chopped parsley or mint (optional). Cover the pie with the other half of the puff pastry. Seal the edges. Cut long slices in the top of the pastry. Mix $^3/_4$ cup milk and 1 egg. Pour on top. Let sit in fridge for one hour before baking. Sprinkle black seed on top. Bake at 350° F. (177° C.) for about 20 minutes.

Variations: Cut pastry into thirds. Layer with pastry, cheese, pastry, cheese and then pastry. Include fried onions and mushrooms with the cheese.

Duqqus
(Eastern Province)

INGREDIENTS

$^1/_2$ tablespoon butter
1 tomato
$1^1/_2$ teaspoons cumin

$^1/_2$ cup chopped onion
$^1/_{16}$ teaspoon red cayenne pepper

Duqqus is often served with kabsa.

Melt $^1/_2$ tablespoon butter with $^1/_2$ cup chopped onion. Grate one tomato and add it to the onion mixture. Add about $^1/_{16}$ teaspoon red pepper and 1-$1^1/_2$ teaspoons cumin. Mix together. Serve.

Matazeez

Munira Al-Ashgar (Dhahran, Eastern Province) (picture page 197)

INGREDIENTS

Dough:
3/4 cup water   1 1/2 cups brown flour
pinch of salt

1 1/2 medium onions, chopped   1/2 kg. meat, chunks
2 hot green peppers   4 cups hot water
2 tablespoons tomato paste   2 whole black limes, poke holes on 2 sides
1 cup eggplant, cut lengthwise into 4-6 pieces
2 tablespoons oil
1 1/2 teaspoons bazaar (mixed spices)   3 tomatoes, diced
salt to taste   2 carrots, cut lengthwise
2 squashes, cut lengthwise into 2-4 pieces
1 cup pumpkin, diced

Add 3/4 cup of water to the flour with a pinch of salt. Knead well and leave aside for half an hour.

Sauté the onions in the oil. Add the meat and the seasoning and two hot green peppers. Cook for three minutes.

Add the tomatoes and cook over medium heat for about 15 minutes, stirring occasionally.

Add four cups of water, salt and tomato paste. Cook until meat is almost done.

While meat is cooking, make dough into small balls the size of a marble.

After placing a small amount of oil in the palm of your hands, take the dough balls and form each into a disc about 2 1/2 inches in diameter.

Add carrots and black lime and cook for 10 minutes. Add squash, then start dropping the *matazeez* (discs) in the hot mixture alternating with pumpkin and eggplant pieces.

Cook for 45 minutes over low heat.

[*Note*: Bazaar is an Arabic mixed spice consisting of coriander, curry, cardamom, black pepper and ginger.]

Faga' Mahmoose (Sautéed Truffles)
Munira Al-Ashgar (Dhahran, Eastern Province)

INGREDIENTS

$^1/_2$ kilogram *faga'* (desert truffles)   water for boiling
2 chopped onions   2 teaspoons oil or butter
spices to taste $^1/_2$ teaspoon cardamom
$^1/_2$ teaspoon black pepper $^1/_2$ teaspoon crushed garlic
4 whole tomatoes or 2 tablespoons tomato paste (optional)

Thoroughly wash the *faga'*. Peel them carefully to prevent sand from sticking to the *faga'*. Soak the *faga'* in cold water for one and a half hours. Cut the *faga'* into one-half-inch cubes and boil in water and salt for one half hour. Then remove the *faga'* from the water.

Fry the onion in the oil until soft. Add the spices and stir. If using tomatoes, add them and cook for ten minutes. Add the *faga'* and cook for one half hour. Serve hot. Makes 2 servings.

Note: *Faga'* are available in Arabian vegetable markets in season. They are also available in cans in some grocery stores.

&a. &a. &a. &a.

Saudi Sambusa
Kamilia Mandoura (Jeddah, Western Province)

INGREDIENTS

Dough:
3 cups flour   3 tablespoons oil
$^1/_2$ teaspoon black seeds   warm water
salt

For the filling:
$^1/_4$ kg ground meat   1 onion
a tablespoon of oil   chopped parsley and boiled eggs (optional)
salt and spices (black pepper, cumin, coriander, galangal)

Add the salt and the black seeds to the flour and mix with the oil. Add the warm water gradually, divide into small balls and leave for $^1/_2$ hour.

Meanwhile, heat the oil. Add the onion and leave for 2 minutes. Add the ground meat and stir until the liquid evaporates, then add spices. Add parsley and chopped boiled eggs if you like. Stuff the dough balls with the filling.

Deep fry them in a hot oil until colour is golden.

Qursan

Kamilia Mandoura (Jeddah, Western Province)

INGREDIENTS

1 large onion, chopped	meat	cubed squash
tomato paste	cumin	black pepper
red pepper	salt	oil
dried lime *(loomi)* powder	cardamom	

qursan bread (available in Mid-Eastern supermarkets especially for this dish)

Add some oil to a hot pan. Add half the onion, leave until gold. Add the meat, stir until water dries. Add the tomato paste, salt and spices. Add some water. Bring to boil and leave until meat is almost cooked. Add the squash and leave until squash is tender. Add water when needed. There should be liquid.

In another pan add a large spoonful of oil and the remaining onion. Leave until golden, then add the ground dried lime, salt, black pepper and cardamom. Fry for a few minutes.

In an oven pan, put a layer of *qursan*, then a layer of the meat and squash, then a layer of the onion mixture, and again repeat the process. Put in oven for 15 minutes

ᶓ ᶓ ᶓ ᶓ

Jarish

Lama A. Khuzayem (Qasim, Central Province)

INGREDIENTS

jarish (crushed wheat)	1 whole chicken
1 dried lime (loomi)	fresh laban (yogurt drink)
brown fried onions	1 lemon, sliced
salt	cumin
cinnamon powder	coriander powder
black pepper	lemon juice

Soak *jarish* in water before cooking. Clean the chicken and boil it whole. Remove the chicken from its broth. Strain it if necessary. Add a whole dried lime, punctured on one side to facilitate seasoning, and then boil the *jarish* in this broth.

Cut the chicken into small pieces and fry it in the spices and lemon juice. After frying, add the chicken and *laban* to the *jarish*. Cook until dry. When serving, top with fried onions.

Aish bi-Laham (Bread with Meat)

Kamilia Mandoura (Jeddah, Western Province)

INGREDIENTS

2 cups flour
1 tablespoon yeast
1 teaspoon sesame

$^1/_4$ cup oil
1 teaspoon black seeds
salt, water

For the filling:
$^1/_4$ kg ground meat
$^1/_4$ bundle of leeks
1 teaspoon black vinegar
1 tablespoon oil
cumin

1 onion
3 tablespoons of tahina
salt and black pepper
1 egg

Mix the dough ingredients together (except the sesame), and add water to form a soft sticky dough. Leave for an hour. Chop the onion. Put oil in a pan. Add onion and stir for 2 minutes, then add the ground meat and stir until all the liquid evaporates. Add salt and spices. Mix tahina with about 3 spoons of water, add the leek after cutting to small pieces, then add vinegar and stir together.

Add the meat to the tahina mixture and stir. Put some oil in a tin, and cover it with the dough. Sprinkle the sesame on the surface. Pour the meat mixture on the top of the dough, put in the oven, at a temperature of about 200° F. (93° C.) and leave for 30 minutes.

Mix the egg and paint the surface with it. Return to oven and leave for about 15 minutes.

🐝 🐝 🐝 🐝

Couscous

INGREDIENTS

2 cups couscous
2 cups water or chicken broth
$^1/_4$ cup olive oil
1 large onion
2 carrots, peeled and diced
1-2 tablespoons butter

$^1/_2$ teaspoon cayenne
1 can chickpeas, drained
$^1/_3$ cup dark seedless raisins
$^1/_3$ cup chopped fresh parsley or mint
2 teaspoons cumin
1 teaspoon cinnamon

Bring water or chicken broth and 1 tablespoon olive oil to a rolling boil. Add couscous. Cover and take off heat. Let stand about 5 minutes until liquid is absorbed. Melt butter in the couscous and then fluff with a fork. Sauté onions and carrots in remaining olive oil for 5-7 minutes. Add spices and stir for one minute. Combine the vegetables and spices with the couscous and serve.

Mufallaq with Meat
Munira Al-Ashgar (Eastern Province)

INGREDIENTS

3 cups *mufallaq* (roasted crushed wheat)   6$^{1}/_{2}$ cups boiling water
salt to taste $^{1}/_{2}$ kg. meat, cut into small pieces
2 large onions, chopped   3 tomatoes, diced
finely ground spices (cinnamon, bazaar, coriander, black lime and cloves)

oil for sautéing

For the garnish:

2 large onions, chopped
$^{1}/_{2}$ teaspoon each finely ground cinnamon, bazaar, coriander, black lemon and cloves
2 tablespoons oil $^{1}/_{2}$ cup cooked chickpeas

In a cooking pot, sauté the onions with the spices. Add the meat and tomatoes and continue stirring. Add the boiling water and cook until the meat is done. Add the *mufallaq* after washing and stir. Let simmer on low heat until the liquid is gone (about 40 minutes).

For the garnish:

In a sauce pan, sauté the onions. Add the spices and stir. Add the chickpeas and stir some more. Put the garnish on top of the *mufallaq* and it is ready to serve.

[*Note*: You can substitute prawns or chicken for meat in the above recipe.]

🐞 🐞 🐞 🐞

Roasted Garlic

Place an entire bulb of garlic in an oven-proof container. Pour in enough olive oil to reach about one quarter of the way up the bulb. Add a cup of water and season with salt, pepper, and herbs, if desired (fresh thyme, oregano, or marjoram, for example). Bake in the oven at 325°F. (163°C.) for one hour.

Hasawi Rice with Shrimp

Munira Al-Ashgar (Dhahran, Eastern Province)

INGREDIENTS

2 cups Hasawi rice $^1/_2$ kg. shrimp, cleaned
1 teaspoon cinnamon   5 cardamom pods
1 teaspoon dried black lime, finely ground
salt to taste   2 large onions, chopped
3 tomatoes, cut medium size   1 tablespoon tomato paste
6 cups water $^1/_2$ cup oil for sautéing
1 tablespoon bazaar (mixed Arabic spices)

Put the onions, the spices and the oil in the cooking pot and sauté until the onion is golden brown. Add the shrimp and stir until browned. Add the tomatoes and the tomato paste, stir and let simmer on medium heat until the tomatoes are soft and most of the liquid is evaporated. Add the water and bring to boil. Add the rice after washing and reduce the heat to low and let it simmer for about 20 minutes. Reduce the heat to very low and let simmer for another 30 minutes.

Note: You can substitute chicken for shrimp in the above recipe.

🐚 🐚 🐚 🐚

A Najdi version of matazeez, p. 192.

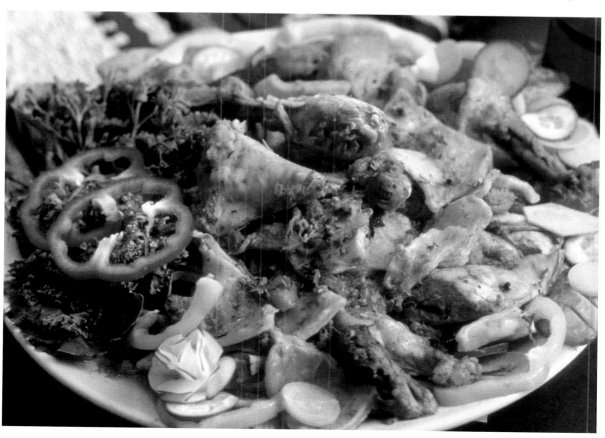

Baked Fennel with Goat's Cheese

INGREDIENTS

2 large fennel bulbs
1 large tomato, sliced
a handful of pine nuts

2 tablespoons olive oil
4 thin rounds of goat's cheese
freshly-ground black pepper to taste.

Cut fennel bulbs in half lengthwise and trim off any small leaves. Drizzle olive oil over both sides and place in a baking dish. Place a thick slice of tomato over each half and bake for 20 minutes at 350° F. (177° C.). Test with a fork to see if the flesh has softened, then place slices of goat cheese on each bulb, cooking for another 10 minutes until the cheese has melted over the fennel and tomato. Remove, then sprinkle with pine nuts and pepper. Serve hot.

🐜 🐜 🐜 🐜

Falafel

INGREDIENTS

2 cups chickpeas
¹/₂ cup parsley, finely chopped
¹/₂ teaspoon cumin
¹/₂ teaspoon pepper

4 onions
1 teaspoon ground coriander
1 teaspoon bicarbonate soda

Soak chickpeas overnight. Remove skins and put chickpeas through a meat grinder with onions and garlic. Grind twice using a fine screen (Alternatives are mashing by hand or using a food processor). Combine with parsley, spices, and soda. Knead well and leave to rest about 30 minutes. Drop by teaspoonful into deep, hot fat and fry until browned on both sides. Drain. Serve hot.

DESSERTS

Anise Cookies
Claudine Shane (USA/Lebanon)

INGREDIENTS

4 cups flour
1 cup oil
1¹/₂ tablespoons anise powder
1¹/₂ cups sugar
1 teaspoon vanilla
grated peel of one lemon

2 eggs
2 tablespoons anise (seed form)
2 tablespoons dry milk
about ¹/₂ cup milk or water
1 teaspoon baking powder

Mix all ingredients. Form into a ball. Take small pieces and roll into snakes. Shape into half-circles or any desired shape. A C-shape is quite popular. Bake 20 minutes at 350° F. (177° C.). Broil for 2 minutes in order to brown the tops.

Baking 20 minutes and broiling for 2 makes a crunchy cookie. For a softer cookie, cook for 18 minutes and broil for 2.

≈ ≈ ≈ ≈

Date Cake
Badria Abahussein (Eastern Province)

INGREDIENTS

2 cups dates
2 teaspoons baking soda
¹/₃ cup sugar
2 teaspoons baking powder

1 cup boiling water
¹/₄ stick butter
2 eggs
1 cup flour

Melt dates in boiling water then add baking soda and butter. Mix in the sugar and eggs and then the flour and baking powder. Bake at 350° F. (177° C.) for 45 minutes. Absolutely delicious!

Date Bars

Munira Al-Ashgar (Eastern Province, Saudi Arabia)

INGREDIENTS

2 ¹/₂ cups flour
¹/₂ cup powdered sugar
1 tablespoon cinnamon
1 cup shortening
1 egg
¹/₂ cup sesame seeds

1 teaspoon baking powder
2 tablespoons *yansoon* (anise)
1 teaspoon nutmeg
2 cups seedless dates
¹/₂ cup evaporated milk

Spices for dates:
1 teaspoon yansoon (anise)   1 teaspoon cinnamon   1 teaspoon nutmeg

Mix all dry ingredients except the sesame seeds and the spices for dates. Add shortening and mix well with fingers.

Add milk and egg. Knead well with fingers. Spread the dough in the bottom of a 9x13x3 in. pan.

Mix the dates with yansoon, cinnamon, nutmeg and half of the sesame seeds. Press lightly in the pan.

Break the remainder of the dough on top of the dates. Sprinkle and press the remaining sesame seeds on top of the mixture. Place in a preheated oven at about 350°F for about 30 minutes. Then place under a broiler until light brown. Cut into one-inch squares and serve.

🐜 🐜 🐜 🐜

Fried Dough Chips with Black Seed

Fatin Hareth (Najran, Southern Province)

INGREDIENTS

1 cup flour
1 teaspoon baking powder
2 tablespoons whole black seed
1 egg
¹/₄ cup oil

5 tablespoons (approximate) of sugar
1 tablespoon yeast
water (about ¹/₂ cup)
1 teaspoon vanilla

Mix all ingredients. Leave for an hour until the dough rises. Roll the dough flat with a rolling pin and cut into small triangles or squares. Fry in oil. Then dip dough chips in *sheerah* or sweet mixture for just less than a minute. Remove, drain and eat immediately!

Sheerah
Fatin Hareth (Najran, Southern Province)

INGREDIENTS

2 cups sugar   1¹/₂ cups water
1 teaspoon vanilla   2 small pieces of lemon peel

This is a sweet mixture to accompany Fried Dough Chips.

Boil ingredients for 10-15 minutes. Dip fried dough chips in this sweet mixture for less than one minute prior to eating.

ʃ. ʃ. ʃ. ʃ.

Kunafa with Banana
Aisha H. Fatany (Makkah, Western Province)

INGREDIENTS

¹/₄ kg *kunafa* (pastry sold by the kilo)   ¹/₂ cup ghee or oil
3 sliced or mashed bananas   *gishta* or cream (optional)
crushed walnuts (optional)

Syrup:

1 cup water   1 cup sugar
1 tablespoon lemon juice   3 teaspoons rose water

Prepare the syrup: Mix water and sugar and heat. When the water starts boiling, then add the lemon juice. Leave until it starts to thicken, then add rose water and leave for two more minutes. Remove from heat and allow to reach room temperature.

Cut *kunafa* 'shoelace' pastry into pieces 1-2 inches in length and mix it well with the ghee. Divide the mixture into two halves. Put the first half in a pan and then put the sliced or mashed bananas on top. Sprinkle some of the walnuts on top of the banana. Add a layer of cream (*gishta*) on top of the banana and walnuts, then add the second layer of *kunafa*. Bake in oven (average temperature) for about 20 minutes or until the top is reddish gold. Pour the syrup on top of the *kunafa* and serve.

Note: Don't pour hot syrup on hot *kunafa*. One of them at least should be cold.

Al-Hesou (Spicy Flour Pudding with Eggs)
(Bahrain)

INGREDIENTS

3 tablespoons rashad (cress seeds)
$1^1/_4$ cups sifted brown flour
$1^1/_4$ cups melted animal fat, ghee, butter or vegetable oil
3 tablespoons al-Hesou spices (*see* spice mixtures)
4-5 cups boiling water
3 eggs, lightly beaten
$1-1^1/_2$ cups sugar

Wash the *rashad* seeds. Soak overnight. Strain and save the water. Dissolve sugar into this water.

Heat one cup of fat in a pot until it begins to steam. Gradually add the flour while stirring until a smooth mixture is obtained. Add the *rashad* and al-Hesou spices. Remove from heat. Add remaining cup of melted fat. Add the sugar solution and half of the water.

Heat again while adding remaining hot water. Stir continuously. A thick smooth batter should form. Boil for five minutes.

Stir in the eggs. Adjust sugar to taste. Partially cover and simmer for ten minutes. Serve hot.

ॐ ॐ ॐ ॐ

Aseeda

INGREDIENTS

2 cups brown flour   2 cups seedless dates
1 cup sugar $^1/_2$ cup ghee
5 cups water   2 tablespoons melted butter
black pepper

Stir flour in a pan over low heat until it turns a light yellow color. Sift and set aside. Place water and dates in a pan and stir on low heat until dates dissolve. Strain.

Mix sugar with ghee. Stir over low heat until golden. Add date mixture and bring to a boil. Then, cool and add half the flour mixture while stirring over low heat. Gradually add remaining ingredients, cover and cook over low heat for 45 minutes.

Serve in individual bowls. Sprinkle with black pepper and dot with butter prior to serving.

SPICE MIXTURES

Al-Hesou Spice Mix

INGREDIENTS

1 cup dried ginger root
1 cup whole black peppercorns
$^1/_3$ cup cinnamon
$^1/_2$ cup cloves
2 tablespoons fenugreek

1 cup cumin
$^1/_2$ cup turmeric
$^1/_2$ cup cardamom
6 whole nutmegs

Mix all ingredients. Grind in an electric grinder or food processor. Store in a dry, airtight glass container.

Fenugreek Paste
(Yemen)

INGREDIENTS

$^1/_4$ cup ground fenugreek
2-4 hot chilis
1 tomato, peeled and chopped
2 cloves garlic, crushed
1 cup finely chopped boiled lamb or chicken
1 cup boiled lentils
1 tablespoon fresh cilantro leaves
bone or chicken stock

1 cup cold water
salt
$^1/_4$ cup chopped onion
$^1/_4$ teaspoon Yemeni spice mix (see p. 204)
1 cup boiled rice
2 tablespoons oil

Soak fenugreek in cold water for five hours. Drain and then beat until frothy. Place in a pot, adding salt and finely chopped chilis (without stalks and seeds). Add remaining ingredients to the pot and blend with just enough stock to moisten. Cook over medium heat, stirring occasionally, while sauce bubbles and thickens. While heating, add more stock as needed. Serve with flat bread.

Yemeni Spice Mix

INGREDIENTS

6 teaspoons black peppercorns
1 teaspoon saffron threads
2 teaspoons turmeric

3 teaspoons caraway seeds
1 teaspoon cardamom seeds

Grind peppercorns, caraway seeds, saffron and cardamom in a blender, or pound in a mortar with a pestle. Stir in powdered turmeric.

Store in an airtight glass jar.

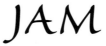

JAM

Middle Eastern Fig Jam

INGREDIENTS

2 pounds dried figs (Turkish, sun-dried, if possible)
1^1/$_2$ pounds granulated sugar
juice of ^{1}/$_2$ lemon
3 tablespoons pine nuts
^{1}/$_4$ teaspoon pulverized mastic

25 ounces water
1 teaspoon ground aniseed
^{1}/$_4$ pound walnuts, chopped

Chop the figs roughly. Boil sugar and water with the lemon juice for a few minutes, then add the figs and simmer gently until they are soft and impregnated with the syrup, which should have thickened enough to coat the back of a spoon. Stir constantly to avoid burning. Add the aniseed, pine nuts and walnuts.

Simmer gently, stirring for a few minutes longer. Remove from the heat and stir the mastic in very thoroughly. (To be properly pulverized, it must have been pounded with sugar.)

Pour into sterilized jars and seal while hot.

DIPS

Baba Ghannouj
(Linda Lebling)

INGREDIENTS

1 large eggplant   1-2 clove(s) garlic
salt to taste   4 tablespoons tahina (sesame paste)
$1/4$ cup water or reserved liquid from cooked eggplant
juice of one lemon, or more to taste

Garnish (optional):
1 tablespoon olive oil   1-2 tablespoons finely chopped parsley
ground sumac (optional)

Grill the whole eggplant over indirect flame on an outdoor barbecue grill (preferred method) or bake it in a 375° F. (190° C.) oven for about 30 minutes, turning once at about the halfway point, until it is very soft on the inside. The grill method imparts a wonderful, slightly smoky flavor to the eggplant, which many prefer.

Let cooked eggplant cool, place it in a bowl and remove the skin carefully, reserving any liquid. Remove seeds to avoid any bitterness (optional). Chop the eggplant finely. In a separate bowl, mash garlic with salt, and add tahina, water or eggplant liquid, and lemon juice, and blend thoroughly. Pour this mixture over the chopped eggplant.

Pound, mash and blend the ingredients with a potato masher or mallet. For finer texture, put the mixture through a blender. Spoon the mixture into a shallow serving dish, garnish the edge with chopped parsley.

Drizzle with olive oil, and sprinkle with a bit of sumac for added lemony tartness.

Serve as a dip with pita bread. This recipe may be doubled or even tripled for larger groups.

🐜 🐜 🐜 🐜

Humous

(Linda Lebling)

INGREDIENTS

1 can (14 $^1/_2$ oz) chickpeas/garbanzo beans $^1/_3$ - $^1/_2$ cup tahina (sesame paste)
$^1/_2$ cup lemon juice (more or less to taste) $^1/_2$ tsp salt (more or less to taste)
1 clove garlic, peeled and crushed (more or less to taste − 3 cloves are wonderful!)
3-5 tablespoon reserved chickpea liquid

Garnish:
1 tablespoon olive oil   2 tablespoons chopped parsley
a handful of reserved whole chickpeas   cumin powder (optional)
paprika (optional)

Drain chickpeas, reserving liquid and a few peas for garnish. Place chickpeas, garlic, tahina, lemon juice and salt in food processor, process to a thick paste. If the mixture is too dry, slowly add one tablespoon at a time of the reserved liquid, until desired consistency. Adjust the flavour to your own liking by adding very small amounts of extra tahina, lemon juice or salt.

Spoon the mixture into a shallow dish.

To garnish, drizzle a little olive oil on top of the humous, sprinkle with parsley and decorate with additional whole chickpeas. Some like to dust the finished product with a little cumin and/or paprika.

Serve as a dip with pita bread.

🐜 🐜 🐜 🐜

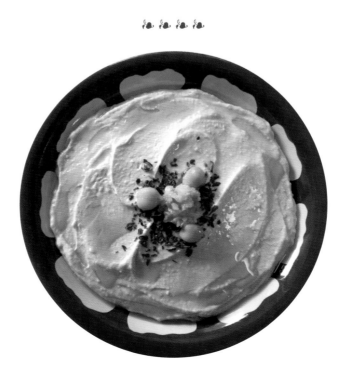

Glossary of Herbal Medicine Terms

Abortifacient – A substance that induces abortion. Also called an **ecbolic**. Example: aloe, *sheeh*.

Alterative – A substance that removes toxins from the body and strengthens the immune system. Once called 'blood cleanser.' Examples: aloe, cinnamon, myrrh, wild rue.

Analgesic – Pain reliever. Examples: chamomile, cinnamon, cloves.

Anesthetic – A substance that reduces or removes sensation.

Anthelmintic – A substance that expels intestinal worms. Also called a **vermifuge**. Examples: *ajwain*, wormwood.

Antibacterial – A substance that suppresses or eliminates bacteria. Example: myrrh.

Antibiotic – A substance that inhibits the growth of or destroys microbes (i.e. bacteria, viruses, yeasts, amoebas).

Antidote – A substance that counteracts poison.

Antiemetic – A substance that prevents nausea or vomiting. Examples: cloves, ginger.

Antifungal – Destroying or preventing the growth of fungi. Example: *neem*.

Anti-inflammatory – Countering or suppressing inflammation. Example: *qaysum*.

Antinauseant – Capable of preventing nausea. Example: perfumed cherry.

Antioxidant – A substance that blocks or inhibits destructive oxidation reactions.

Antiputrefactive, Antiputrescent – Countering or protecting from putrefaction; antiseptic. Example: myrrh.

Antipyretic – A substance that lowers fever. Also called a **febrifuge** or **refrigerant**. Example: *qaysum*.

Antiseptic – A substance that inhibits growth of microorganisms. Example: aloe, sage.

Antiscorbutic – a substance that counteracts scurvy, a disease caused by lack of vitamin C in the diet.

Antispasmodic – A substance that prevents or relieves convulsions or spasms. Examples: basil, chamomile, myrrh, sage.

Antiviral – Destroying or preventing the growth of viruses. Example: neem.

Aphrodisiac – Something that increases generative tissue substance (tonic) or increases the functioning of reproductive organs (stimulant). Examples: fenugreek, hibiscus, *tarthuth*.

Aromatic – A substance with a fragrant smell. Example: frankincense

Astringent – A substance that causes tissues to contract, sometimes restricting blood or mucus flow. Usually applied topically. Example: *tarthuth*.

Cardiotonic – Having a positive or tonic effect on the heart. Example: milkweed.

Carminative – A substance that controls intestinal gas or flatulence. Examples: chamomile, fennel, lime, peppermint, ajwain, basil, cardamom, cinnamon, ginger.

Cataplasm – A soft, moist substance, such as meal or clay, spread on a cloth and applied to the skin to counter an infection or improve circulation. Also known as a **poultice**.

Cathartic – A laxative, or medicine that causes evacuation of the bowels. Also called a **purgative**. Examples: senna, aloe.

Cholagogue – A substance that stimulates bile flow into the intestine. Examples: senna, qaysum.

Collyrium – Pl. collyria. A medicinal lotion applied to the eyes. An eyewash.

Decoction – An extract obtained by boiling a plant in water and straining the resulting liquid.

Demulcent – A substance that relieves irritation of the lining of the stomach, bladder and other organs.

Detersive – cleansing (substance).

Depurative – Purifying; purgative.

Diaphoretic – A substance that promotes perspiration and thereby counters fever, muscle aches, etc. Examples: basil, *ajwain*, cardamom, cinnamon, ginger, chamomile, fennel.

Diluent – A substance used to dilute another substance. An agent used to dilute the blood.

Diuretic – An agent that promotes urination. Example: *qaysum*.

Dysmenorrhea – Painful menstrual cramps.

Ecbolic – See **abortifacient**.

Electuary – Ingredients mixed with honey or syrup to form a paste. Example: fenugreek, black seed.

Emetic – An agent that causes vomiting. Also called a **vomitive**. Example: wild rue.

Emmenagogue – A substance that brings on or increases menstruation. Examples: chamomile, aloe, hibiscus, rose.

Emollient – A substance that softens or soothes the skin. Example: oils.

Expectorant – That which prompts bronchial secretions and helps to eject them. Examples: ginger, cardamom, cinnamon, cloves, sage, thyme.

Febrifuge – See **antipyretic**.

Galactogogue – A substance that increases secretion of breast milk. Examples: cumin, fennel, nettle.

Gastric – Having to do with the stomach.

Hypertensive – Marked by increased blood pressure.

Hypotensive – Marked by reduced blood pressure.

Infusion – A liquid produced by steeping a substance in water.

Menorrhagia – Excessive uterine bleeding at regular times of menstruation.

Mucilaginous – Resembling or characteristic of mucilage: soft, slimy, sticky.

Narcotic – A drug that produces sleep or general anesthesia.

Nervine – Having the ability to act upon or affect the nerves; quieting nervous excitement. A tonic with this quality. Example: lemon balm.

Oxidation – A chemical reaction in which oxygen reacts with another substance, resulting in a chemical change, often some type of deterioration or spoilage.

Oxymel – A mixture of honey, water, vinegar and spice, boiled to a syrup.

Poultice – See **cataplasm**.

Purgative – See **cathartic**.

Refrigerant – See **antipyretic**.

Rubefacient – A mild irritant that reddens the skin. Example: ginger.

Soporific – A substance that produces sleep.

Stimulant – A substance that increases physiological activity, especially of an organ. Examples: fennel, anise.

Stomachic – A substance that improves digestion and the appetite. Examples: cardamom, cumin, ginger, perfumed cherry, turmeric.

Styptic (haemostatic) – A substance that, applied topically, checks bleeding. Example: *tarthuth*.

Tonic – An agent that helps improve the general system of the human body, restoring normal tone. Example: aloe.

Vermifuge – See **anthelmintic**.

Vomitive – See **emetic**.

Vulnerary – A healing substance used to treat cuts and wounds, often as a poultice. Examples: aloe, turmeric.

Index of Common Ailments

Antibiotic
Myrrh

Appetite, loss of
Coffee
Dates

Asthma
Black seed
Honey

Bleeding
Alum

Blood Cleanser
Arugula
Cress

Boils and Abscesses
Cress
Mangrove

Bones
Black Seed
Cress
Fenugreek
Frankincense

Breast Abscesses and Mastitis
Fenugreek

Breastfeeding
Caraway
Fenugreek
Nakhwa

Bruises
Dates
Turmeric

Burns & Sunstroke
Dates
Henna
Honey

Myrrh
Powdered pomegranate peelings
Turmeric

Chest Complaints
Frankincense
Myrrh

Chicken Pox
Henna

Childbirth (*Note:* Treatments for strengthening or cleansing a mother are generally followed during the 40 days after childbirth.)
Alum
Anise
Arta
Black seed
Cardamom
Chamomile
Cinnamon
Cress
Cumin
Dates
Fenugreek
Fresh soup
Ginger
Honey
Incense
Julab
Frankincense (*Laban thakr*)
Myrrh
Red seed
Saffron

Cholesterol
Ginger

Colds or Coughs
Anise
Asafoetida
Basil
Black Seed
Chamomile

Cloves
Cumin
Frankincense
Garlic
Ginger
Honey
Myrrh
Tahina
Thyme
Turmeric

Colic
Anise
Caraway
Chamomile
Cumin
Dates
Fennel
Lime, Dried
Mint
Myrrh

Constipation
Arugula

Cuts or Wounds
Alum
Arugula
Basil
Cloves
Coffee
Fenugreek
Frankincense
Garlic
Henna
Honey
Myrrh
Onion Skin
Sarcocol
Tarthuth
Toothpaste
Turmeric

Diabetes
Aloe
Alum
Arta
Fenugreek
Frankincense
Germander
Myrrh
Wormwood *(sheeh)*

Diarrhoea
Arugula
Banana
Dates
Garlic
Ginger
Honey
Lime, Dried
Myrrh
Thyme

Eyes
Cloves
Coffee
Cucumber
Ginger
Rose
Turmeric

Fatigue
Arugula
Cinnamon
Dates
Fenugreek
Garlic
Honey
Onions

Fevers
Arugula
Henna
Mahaleb Cherry

Flatulence (Intestinal Gas)
Arta
Caraway
Cardamom
Cumin
Fennel
Incense *(bukhoor)*
Lavender
Mint
Myrrh
Rose
Thyme

Hair Loss
Aloe
Arugula
Black Seed
Castor Oil
Henna
Onion
Sidr

Headaches
Black Seed
Cloves
Coffee
Ginger
Henna
Mint
Myrrh
Onion
Petroleum
Sidr

Heart Trouble
Black Seed
Chamomile
Garlic
Rose
Saffron

High Blood Pressure
Hibiscus

Indigestion
Anise
Arugula
Castor Oil
Chamomile
Coriander
Cucumber
Cumin
Date
Frankincense
Honey
Mint
Myrrh
Nakhwa
Pomegranate
Sarcocol
Wormwood *(sheeh)*

Infections
Arugula
Frankincense
Henna
Myrrh
Turmeric

Insect Bites and Stings
Basil
Dates
Garlic

Insect Repellant
Wormwood *(Bu'aythiran)*

Insomnia
Anise
Black Seed
Honey
Mint
Rose
Wormwood *(Bu'aythiran)*
Yogurt

Intestinal Worms
Honey

Joint Pain
Date

Kidneys
Black Seed
Cress
Hibiscus
Wormwood *(sheeh)*

Liver
Cardamom
Cumin
Fenugreek
Frankincense
Honey
Thyme

Lungs
Frankincense

Measles
Henna

Memory
Frankincense

Menstrual Pain
Anise
Chamomile
Cinnamon
Cumin
Fenugreek
Frankincense
Lemon Balm
Lime, Dried
Myrrh
Parsley
Sage

Nausea
Cloves
Coffee
Dates
Frankincense
Ginger

Newborn Care
Dates
Fenugreek
Sarcocol

Obesity
Sage

Oedema
Germander

Oral Care
Arak
Frankincense
Neem
Walnut Bark

Purgative
Aloe
Germander

Rheumatism
Black Seed
Dates
Wormwood *(Bu'aythiran)*

Sexual Vigor
Arugula

Sinus Congestion
Pomegranate

Skin Ailments
Arta
Turmeric

Sore Throats
Clove
Ginger
Honey
Lemon
Myrrh
Petroleum
Sage

Stomach Pain
Anise
Black Seed
Chamomile
Cinnamon
Coffee
Cumin
Dates
Fenugreek
Frankincense
Garlic
Ginger
Honey
Lime, Dried
Mint
Myrrh
Petroleum
Sage

Thyme
Wormwood *(sheeh)*
Yarrow

Stomach Ulcers
Arta
Pomegranate
Tarthuth

Stress
Anise
Basil
Chamomile

Toothache, Tonsil and Larynx Pain
Asafoetida
Anise
Cloves
Black Seed

Vomiting
Dates
Garlic

Warts
Garlic
Purslane

Bibliography & References

Abdoh, Othman Labib, and Azer Armanious. *The Medical Botanical Vocabulary from Arabic into English, French and Latin*. Cairo: Misr Press, 1929.

Abercrombie, Thomas J. 'Arabia's Frankincense Trail.' *National Geographic*, Vol. 168, No. 4. (Oct. 1985): 474-513.

AWA (American Women of Amman). *Sahtain Wa Hana Cookbook*. Amman: National Press, 1992.

Barreveld, W.H. *Date Palm Products*. FAO Agricultural Products Bulletin No. 101. Rome: Food and Agriculture Organization of the United Nations, 1993.

Basson, Philip W., and Lisa Bobrowski. *Biotopes of the Western Arabian Gulf: Marine Life and Environments of Saudi Arabia*. Dhahran, Saudi Arabia: Aramco Dept. of Loss Prevention and Environmental Affairs, 1977.

Batanouny, K.H., in collaboration with S. Abou Tabi, M. Shabana and F. Soliman. *Wild Medicinal Plants in Egypt: An Inventory to Support Conservation and Sustainable Use*. Cairo: Academy of Scientific Research and Technology, Egypt, and International Union for Conservation (IUCN), 1999.

Beardwood, Mary. *The Children's Encyclopaedia of Arabia*. London: Stacey International, 2001.

Bedevian, Armenag K. *Illustrated Polyglottic Dictionary of Plant Names*. Cairo: Argus & Papazian Presses, 1936.

Bilkadi, Zayn. 'Ancient Oil Industries.' Parts 1-3. *Aramco World*, July-August 1994, January-February 1995 and September-October 1995.

Blatter, Ethelbert. *Flora Arabica*. Records of the Botanical Survey of India, Vol. VIII, Nos. 1-4. Calcutta: Superintendent Government Printing, India, 1919.

Bown, Deni. *Encyclopedia of Herbs and Their Uses*. New York: DK Publishing, 1995.

Brinker, Francis J. *Herb Contraindication and Drug Interactions*. Sandy, Ore.: Eclectic Medical Publications, 1998.

Burckhardt, John Lewis. *Travels in Arabia*. London: Henry Colburn, 1829.

Burton, Richard F. *Personal Narrative of a Pilgrimage to El-Medinah and Mecca*. London: Longman, Brown, Green, and Longmans, 1855-56.

Chapman, Pat. *Pat Chapman's Curry Bible*. London: Hodder & Stoughton, 1998.

Chevallier, Andrew. *Encyclopedia of Medicinal Plants*. London: Dorling Kindersley, 2001.

Clevely, A., K. Richmond, S. Morris and L. Mackley. *Herbs & Spices: A Cook's Bible*. New York: Lorenz Books, 2000.

Collenette, Sheila. *Wildflowers of Saudi Arabia*. Riyadh: National Commission for Wildlife Conservation and Development, 1999.

Coombes, Allen J. *Dictionary of Plant Names*. Portland, Ore.: Timber Press, 1986.

Cornes, M.D. and C.D. *The Wild Flowering Plants of Bahrain: An Illustrated Guide*. London: Immel Publishing, 1989.

Dalby, Andrew. *Dangerous Tastes: The Story of Spices*. London: British Museum Press, 2000.

Dickson, Violet. *The Wild Flowers of Kuwait and Bahrain*. London: Allen & Unwin, 1955.

Dols, Michael W., trans. *Medieval Islamic Medicine: Ibn Ridwan's Treatise 'On the Prevention of Bodily Ills in Egypt.'* Berkeley, Calif.: University of California Press, 1984.

Doughty, Charles. *Travels in Arabia Deserta*. London: Jonathan Cape, 1924.

Duke, James A. *Herbs of the Bible: 2000 Years of Plant Medicine*. Loveland: Interweave Press, 1999.

Elliott, Jeri. *Your Door to Arabia*. Invercargill, New Zealand: Craig Printing Co. Ltd., 1992.

El Qassani, A. S. *Dhofar: The Land of Frankincense*. Ruwi, Oman: International Printing Press, 1984.

Feeney, John. 'Desert Truffles Galore.' *Saudi Aramco World*, September/October 2002.
—— 'The Red Tea of Egypt.' *Saudi Aramco World*, September/October 2001.

Felter, Harvey W., and John U. Lloyd. *King's American Dispensatory*. 2 vols. 18th edition. Third revision: Cincinnatti, Ohio: Ohio Valley Co., 1898.

Ghazanfar, Shahina A. *Handbook of Arabian Medicinal Plants*. Boca Raton, Florida: CRC Press, 1994.

Gladstar, Rosemary. *The Science and Art of Herbology*. E. Barre, Vt.: Sage Publications, n.d.

Golding, Julia A. *The Benefits of the Use of Stinging Nettles in Herbal Preparations*. Master Herbalist thesis. Springfield, Utah: School of Natural Healing, 2001.

Grieve, Mrs. M. *A Modern Herbal*. New York: Harcourt, Brace & Co., 1931.

Guest, Evan, with assistance from Ali Al-Rawi. *Flora of Iraq. Vol. 1: Introduction to the Flora*. Baghdad: Ministry of Agriculture, 1966.

Hansen, Eric. The Beekeepers of Wadi Du'an. *Saudi Aramco World*, January/February 1995.

Harrison, R.H. *Healing Herbs of the Bible*. Leiden: E.J. Brill, 1966.

Hayward, Michael R. 'The Roses of Taif.' *Saudi Aramco World*, November/December 1997.

Heinerman, John. *Miracle Healing Herbs*. Paramus, N.J.: Prentice Hall, 1998.

Hooper, David. *Useful Plants and Drugs of Iran and Iraq.* Botanical Series, Field Museum of Natural History, Vol. 9, No. 3. Chicago: Field Museum, 1937.

Jabbur, Jibrail S. *The Bedouins and the Desert: Aspects of Nomadic Life in the Arab East.* Translated by Lawrence I. Conrad. Albany: State University of New York Press, 1995.

Jordan, Michele Anna. 'Making the Most of Garlic.' *Kitchen Gardener*, No. 19. (February/March 1999):24-28.

Al-Kahtani, J.S.M., M.A. Al-Yahya and I.A. Al-Meshal. *Medicinal Plants of Saudi Arabia.* Vols. I and II. Riyadh: King Saud University, 2000.

Kamal, Hassan. *Encyclopaedia of Islamic Medicine.* Cairo: General Egyptian Book Organization, 1975.

Karim, Fawzi M., and Saleh A. Quraan. *Medicinal Plants of Jordan.* Irbid: Yarmouk University, 1986.

Kloss, Jethro. *Back to Eden.* Loma Linda: Back to Eden Books, 1981.

Kopf, L., trans. and ed., and F. S. Bodenheimer, ed. *The Natural History Section from a 9th Century 'Book of Useful Knowledge': The 'Uyun al-Akhbar of Ibn Qutayba.* Paris: Academie Internationale d'Histoire des Sciences, 1949.

Krueger, Haven C. *Avicenna's Poem on Medicine.* Springfield, Ill.: Charles C. Thomas, 1963.

Lebling, Robert W. 'The Treasures of Tarthuth.' *Saudi Aramco World*, March/April 2003.

Levey, Martin. *Early Arabic Pharmacology: An Introduction Based on Ancient and Medieval Sources.* Leiden: E.J. Brill, 1973.
——, trans. and ed. *The Medical Formulary or Aqrabadhin of Al-Kindi: Translated with a Study of its Materia Medica.* Madison, Wisc.: University of Wisconsin Press, 1966.
——, and Noury Al-Khaledy. *The Medical Formulary of Al-Samarqandi.* Philadelphia: University of Pennsylvania Press, 1967.

Lewis, W.H., and M.P.F. Elvin-Lewis. *Medical Botany.* New York: John Wiley & Sons, 1977.

Lipscombe Vincett, Betty A. *Golden Days in the Desert: Wild Flowers of Saudi Arabia.* London: Immel Publishing, 1984.
—— *Wild Flowers of Central Saudi Arabia.* Milan: Pi. Me. Editrice, 1977.

Mallos, Tess. *The Complete Middle East Cookbook.* Riyadh: Jarir Bookstore, 1996.

Mandaville, James P. *Flora of Eastern Saudi Arabia.* London: Kegan Paul International Jointly with the National Commission for Wildlife Conservation and Development, Riyadh: 1990.
—— *Wild Flowers of Northern Oman.* London: Bartholomew Books, 1978.

Mauger, Thierry. *Undiscovered Asir.* London: Stacey International, 1993.

Migahid, Ahmad Mohammad. *Flora of Saudi Arabia.* Fourth Edition. 3 Vols. Riyadh: King Saud University, 1996.

Miller, A.G. 'The genus Lavandula in Arabia and Tropical NE Africa.' *Notes Royal Botanic Garden Edinburgh*, 1985,. 42(3):503-528

Miller, A.G., and Miranda Morris. *Plants of Dhofar: The Southern Region of Oman: Traditional, Economic and Medicinal Uses.* Muscat: The Office of the Advisor for Conservation of the Environment, Diwan of the Royal Court, Sultanate of Oman, 1988.

Ministry of Information, State of Bahrain. *Bahrain National Museum.* London: Immel Publishing Ltd., 1993.

Morris, Miranda. 'The Soqotra Archipelago: concepts of good health and everyday remedies for illness.' *Proceedings of the Seminar for Arabian Studies* 33 (2003); 319-341.

Musil, Alois. *Arabia Deserta: A Topographical Itinerary, Expedition of 1908-09.* N.Y.: American Geographical Society, 1927.

Nawwab, Ni'mah I. 'The Culinary Kingdom.' *Aramco World*, January/February 1999.

Palgrave, William Gifford. *Personal Narrative of a Year's Journey Through Central and Eastern Arabia (1862-63).* London: Macmillan and Co., 1883.

Parfitt, J., and S. Valentine. *Dates.* Oman: Dateflake Co., 1995.

Pepperdine, Donna. *Natural Remedies of Saudi Arabia.* Master Herbalist thesis. Burnaby, Canada: Dominion Herbal College, 2002.

Potter, G., and R. Wellington. *Lehi in the Wilderness.* Springville, UT: Cedar Fort, Inc. 2003.

Rodinson, Maxime, A.J. Arberry and Charles Perry, translators. *Medieval Arab Cookery.* Devon, U.K.: Prospect Books, 2001.

Salloum, H. J. Peters. *From the Lands of Figs and Olives.* New York: Interlink Books, 2002.

Al-Saud, Noura bint Muhammad; Al-Jawharah Muhammad Al-'Anqari; and Madeha Muhammad Al-'Ajroush. *Abha: Bilad Asir, South-Western Region of the Kingdom of Saudi Arabia.* Riyadh: 1989.

Simon, J.E., A.F. Chadwick and L.E. Craker. *Herbs: An Indexed Bibliography. 1971-1980. The Scientific Literature on Selected Herbs, and Aromatic and Medicinal Plants of the Temperate Zone.* Hamden, Conn.: Archon Books, 1984.

Skipwith, Ashkahain. *Ashkahain's Saudi Cooking of Today.* London: Stacey International, 1986.

Symonds, Alexia. 'Pomegranates: Aphrodite's Aphrodisiac.' *Sun Jet: Cyprus Airways In-Flight Magazine.* (Winter 2000/2001): 50-55.

Al Taie, Lamees Abdullah. *Al-Azaf: The Omani Cookbook.* Ruwi, Oman: Oman Bookshop LLC., 1995.

Thesiger, Wilfred. *Arabian Sands.* New York: E.P. Dutton, 1959.

United Nations Educational, Scientific and Cultural Organization (UNESCO). *Medicinal Plants of the Arid Zones.* Paris: UNESCO, 1960.

Vidal, F.S. *The Oasis of al-Hasa.* New York: Arabian American Oil Company, 1955.

Walker, John, trans. *Folk Medicine in Modern Egypt: Being the Relevant Parts of the Tibb al-Rukka or Old Wives' Medicine of 'Abd al-Rahman Isma'il*. London: Luzac & Co., 1934.

Wallin, Georg August. *Travels in Arabia (1845 and 1848)*. Cambridge, England: Falcon-Oleander, 1979.

Watt, Martin, and Wanda Sellar. *Frankincense and Myrrh*. Saffron Walden: The C.W. Daniel Company, Ltd., 1996.

Wilcox, Edie. 'The Herbal Waters of Bahrain.' *Bahrain Confidential*. (September 2003):44-45.

Zand, Kamal Hafuth, and John A. and Ivy E. Videan, trans. *The Eastern Key: Kitab al-Ifadah wa'l-I'tibar of 'Abd al-Latif al-Baghdadi*. London: George Allen and Unwin Ltd., 1965.

Al Zayani, Afnan Rashid. *A Taste of the Arabian Gulf*. Bahrain: Oriental Press, 1988.

Zohary, Michael. *Geobotanical Foundations of the Middle East*. Stuttgart: Gustav Fischer Verlag, 1973.

Websites:

Classic Herbal Texts Online: http://www.ibiblio.org/herbmed/eclectic/main.html

Dioscorides' Materia Medica (German): http://www.tiscalinet.ch/materiamedica/

Donna Pepperdine's Herbal Educator: http://www.herbaleducator.com/

Dr. James Duke's Phytochemical and Ethnobotanical Databases: http://www.ars-grin.gov/duke/

Famine Foods Database by Robert (Bob) L. Freedman:
http://www.hort.purdue.edu/newcrop/FamineFoods/ff_home.html

Gernot Katzer's Spice Pages: http://webdb.uni-graz.at/~katzer/engl/

HerbMed Herbal Database: http://www.herbmed.org/

Heritage of Bahrain: http://www.geocities.com/z52264159/5-Heritage.htm

King's American Dispensatory: http://www.ibiblio.org/herbmed/eclectic/kings/main.html

Latifa School for Girls (UAE) Islamic Medicine Website:
http://www.lsg.sch.ae/departments/history/arabic_medicine_web/index.htm

Medicinal, Culinary and Aromatic Plants in the Near East:
http://www.fao.org/docrep/X5402e/x5402e00.htm

Robert Lebling's Handbook of Arabian Medicinal Herbs:
http://www.geocites.com/eyeclaudius.geo/HERBALME.htm

Index by Latin Name

Index by Arabic Name

(Readers are referred to the individual entry for other Arabic names)